You Can't Just Eat a Cheeseburger:

How to thrive through eating disorder recovery

By Justine Duppong, MS, MHA

With contributions from

Carolyn Costin, MFT, M.A., M.Ed.

Keesha Broome, M.A., MFT

Doris Smeltzer

Barbara Truitt, RD, LD/N

ISBN:0615811884
ISBN-13:9780615811888

DEDICATION

To my adorable husband—the perfect match to my heart, mind, and soul.

CONTENTS

ACKNOWLEDGMENTS

This book project never would have become anything more than a dream without the continued contributions, support, and encouragement of the hundred or so people I corresponded with over the past six years of its completion. Although I was not able to include quotes from every person who shared insight, a list of each person who contributed may be found at the back of this book. To each one of you, I will be forever grateful. Because of each one of you, I will be forever inspired.

A special thank you to Carolyn Costin, Keesha Broome, Doris Smeltzer, and Barbara Truitt, for believing in this project enough to take time out of your busy schedules and share your professional viewpoints. Thank you to my enthusiastic team of editors, including especially Laura Geilanfeldt, Doris Smeltzer, and of course that perpetual source of wisdom, my Pops.

Thank you to countless friends and family members who have encouraged me in multiple ways over the years (Mom, even if you are wholly biased, you are the best cheerleader anyone could ever ask for!).

Thank you, my wonderful husband Todd, for always believing in me, supporting me, and challenging me to grow intellectually, emotionally, and spiritually. You are my best friend, and I love overanalyzing the world (and beyond) with you. Thank you for showing me what true and unconditional love is really like.

Thank you St. Anthony, St. Joseph, and our Blessed Mother, for your constant love and intercession, and for serving as perfect examples of true faith.

Dear Heavenly Father, thank you for the great mercy and graces you have provided me, no matter how undeserving I have always been. I cannot look back and find a moment of my life when you were not there to guide me—even in the years when I thought that I for some reason knew better than you what I needed. Thank you for never giving up on me.

Introduction
How (and why) it all began

If you struggle with disordered eating, an exercise disorder, or poor body image, you've probably wondered: Is it really possible to "just eat" what you want, without becoming overweight? How are you supposed to eat "normally" if you go out to a restaurant? What do you say to the person you're dating about your eating habits? How do you stop obsessing about food, your exercise routine, and your body? How can you start working *with* what you've got, instead of against it?

A few years ago, I found myself searching for my own answers. I was five years into an eating disorder, and I wasn't sure who I could talk to about it. Even after reading practically every eating disorder-related book I could get my hands on, I still had unanswered questions. Rather than giving up, I set out to find real people who could answer all of the random questions I had about recovery.

For over three years I scoured internet forums and recovery websites, wrote countless emails, and made phone calls to anyone I thought might be able to help. I created a list of over a hundred insightful people, from everyday men and women in recovery, to professionals in the eating disorder treatment field—all who actually took time to answer literally *pages* of questions from me!

It's often said that a project is worth your time if you can help just one person with it. Well if that's so, then this book was a success long before it was published—because it saved *me.* I suffered from bulimia for three years, and anorexia for a period of time after that—all because I couldn't quite figure out "how" to recover. In some of my darkest, loneliest moments, it was the encouragement and insight I received from the people I connected with throughout this project that gave me the hope and focus I needed in order to reach my own goals.

In this book I'll share some of the common themes I discovered throughout both my own recovery and my interactions with all those people, so as to give you a comprehensive picture of what it takes to *really* heal from disordered eating and body image. Even if you don't meet all of the criteria for having a clinically-diagnosed eating disorder, this book will help you transform the way you view your diet, body, relationships, and life. It's a self-help guide and mini workbook in one, all wrapped up in my own story: Within each chapter you'll find tips for every aspect of the process, as well as how to overcome some of the roadblocks you might face along the way. Toward the end of each chapter you'll find goal-oriented journal questions, followed by a special section for your loved ones with tips, questions they can ask you, and journal questions of their own. Each chapter concludes with a special "Q & A" section filled with advice from field experts: Author, advocate, and parent Doris Smeltzer; author, therapist, and eating disorders specialist Carolyn Costin; therapist Keesha Broome; and eating disorders dietitian Barbara Truitt.

My aim throughout this book is to help you "upcycle" your whole life: What do I mean by that? If you've never heard the word before, in the Do-It-Yourself world, the term "upcycle" basically means to take something old or unusable and turn it into something of value that *works* for you. It's kind of like recycling, with a twist: For example, you can upcycle an old wine bottle by decorating it and turning it into a pretty vase, or you can make a funky coaster out of an empty soda can. Now, I'm not actually telling you to start collecting people's old stuff and turning it into things to sell on ebay, because that would be an entirely different book (although it might not be a bad idea!). I take the concept of upcycling and apply it directly to your life. That means adapting the way you think, feel, and act, in a way that will help you finally get out of your self-defeating rut and start creating the life of your dreams.

Upcycling is a simple way to apply concepts associated with Cognitive Behavioral Therapy (CBT). If you're not familiar with CBT, it's a therapeutic approach that emphasizes the relationship between thoughts, feelings, and actions. It is believed that our thoughts influence our feelings, which thereby influence our behaviors. If you think something negative, you're probably not going to feel very good. If you're not feeling good, you might not make the best decisions. If, on the other hand, you have a positive thought that creates a good feeling, you're much more likely to act in a positive way. CBT has been used to effectively treat all kinds of mental illnesses, such as anxiety, depression, and of course, eating disorders.

Please note that my interpretation of some of the principles behind Cognitive Behavioral Therapy do not encompass every aspect of CBT and are not a substitute for professional help—they are simply guidelines to help you start working on some key areas. Throughout this book I'll help you not only upcycle and improve your thoughts, feelings, and behaviors, but also take a look at specific areas of your life—like your relationships, eating and exercise habits, and how you spend your time—where you can make effective changes that will transform your whole experience.

I'm living proof that upcycling can have some truly wonderful results. Today, instead of remaining trapped in a destructive cycle, I am living the kind of life I always envisioned: I'm doing the things I've always dreamed of doing, I'm married to my best friend and true love, and I'm finally genuinely *happy*. My new life didn't come from achieving a certain weight, or trying to change myself somehow; rather, it came from discovering and embracing who I already am. That process is the essence of recovery, and throughout this book, I hope to guide you in figuring it out for yourself.

What would your life look like if you could free yourself from debilitating thoughts about food and your body? What kinds of things do you dream of achieving? How can you begin to open up your whole world, right now?

Your life is waiting for you—so what are you waiting for?

1 Set Your Table:
Building the foundation for recovery

"Nobody can go back and start a new beginning, but anyone can start today and make a new ending."

--Maria Robinson

"Mom? Do you think I'm going crazy?"

My mother looked at me from across the car in the parking lot outside my apartment, her mouth hanging slightly open in surprise for a moment before she responded. "What? Honey, of course not."

I felt the fluttering, bubbling fear begin to take over my body again. My heart felt about six times its normal size as it beat against my chest. My hands were sweating. I shivered and tried to stop my teeth from chattering as I spoke again. "He…he told me I'm going crazy and that I'm all screwed up. He said we'd have to send me away somewhere because I'm never going to get better."

The last time he had said that to me had been about a week ago, during one of our fights. That day, he had been standing over me and yelling, while I lay on the cold kitchen floor, my body curled up into a tight little cocoon.

I grasped the door handle as my surroundings began to spin again; patches of darkness danced with splotches of color through my field of vision.

"I'm so scared, Mom. Mom, I'm so scared…" A rancid sick feeling swelled up into my stomach as I thought about how I had left work an hour ago. I had been on the floor behind my desk, my feet up on my chair, terrified I was going to pass out. Over the past few weeks I had been experiencing an onslaught of panic attacks, as my fights with him got progressively worse. It was hard for me to sleep at night, as I thought about how different my life was from what I'd always envisioned for myself when I was younger: I'd always imagined that I'd be married to some wonderful guy after college, with one or two adorable little curly-haired, bright-eyed kids, and a big house in the country (picket fence optional). I thought I'd have a great job, lots of friends, and be very happy. I'd probably have shiny blonde hair, perfectly-manicured nails, and a bright red sports car or something, too. I don't know.

Life doesn't always end up like you think it will. The summer after I turned 24, I wasn't working in a backyard vegetable garden or painting the walls of a nursery with my storybook husband. I was curled up between my mom and dad on their sofa, empty and quivering. After six years of being with someone so horribly wrong for me, I'd abandoned all hope of ever finding real love and starting a family. I felt so messed up inside that I wasn't sure I'd ever be able to hold any sort of job again, let alone get out of my parents' house. In high school I had been the girl everyone thought was going to really do something with her life—and now, it felt like it was all just shattered in little jagged pieces around me.

So what the heck happened?

I've often heard it said that although not every diet leads to an eating disorder, every eating disorder begins with a diet. My downward spiral started with my first diet, during my freshman year of high school. By the time I was a junior, that diet had gradually evolved into bulimia. My fixation on food and my body became a way for me to avoid dealing with some of the fears and worries I had about life.

When I went off to college a year and a half later, I jumped right into a relationship with the first person I met. All of a sudden, I was dating a cocky football player who had come all the way across the country on a big scholarship. I didn't know anything about him, but I missed my family horribly, and the friends that I was living with all seemed to forget I existed as soon as we all set foot on campus. As lonely and insecure as I was, I thought a relationship would give me some sort of validation. Beyond that, I was terrified of the potential damage the bulimia was doing to my body. It scared me to be away from my family for the first time, knowing that something horrible might happen without having anyone around to help me. It made me feel safer to have someone nearby, "just in case"—even if that somebody wasn't anybody I would have ever hung out with in high school. Together, the eating disorder and that relationship numbed every glimmer of my old personality, and ate away every last little shred of my confidence. It was only a matter of time before I knew I would never be able to survive as long as I continued to hold onto either one of them.

Like me, you may be aware of habits or relationships in your own life that are destroying your chances at health and happiness. My aim throughout this book is to show you not only how to recover from an eating disorder, but also how to "upcycle" your life, by recreating your relationships, thoughts, feelings, and actions (if you haven't already, please see this book's introduction for more on my definition of upcycling). It truly is amazing how just a few straightforward changes can transform your entire existence!

As you probably know, the first step to making any change is realizing that a change needs to be made. If you're anything like I was, you might be really good at coming up with justifications for some of your "weird" or obsessive habits. However, it's those "harmless" habits that are keeping you stuck in a sad, stagnant, and destructive rut.

Is your life in need of some serious upcycling? The following is a checklist you can use to evaluate some of your food and body-related thoughts and behaviors:

How do you know if some of your habits are disordered?

Do you:

- Avoid eating with other people or eating at restaurants?
- Spend a significant amount of time thinking about food, exercise, or your body?
- Worry excessively about your body composition, how much you weigh, or how your clothes are fitting?
- Weigh yourself multiple times throughout the day?
- Frequently "check" the appearance of certain parts of your body to evaluate their size or leanness/"fatness?"
- Constantly count calories, fat grams, or other food-related numbers?
- Avoid eating certain foods or food groups entirely, because you are afraid of what they might "do" to your body?
- Avoid eating foods you once loved?
- Refuse to take even a bite or two of something that isn't in your "plan" for the day?
- Eat the same foods every day, without variation?
- Feel anxious or tense about eating?
- Feel guilty or ashamed after eating?
- Have anxiety about the physical feelings associated with eating (bloating, fullness, etc.)?
- Spend a great deal of time looking at recipes or cooking for other people, without trying any of the things you make yourself?
- Ever feel "out of control" while eating, or worry that you won't be able to stop if you allow yourself to eat normally?
- Eat until you feel sick?
- Cut your food into tiny pieces?
- Hide food under your plate or in your napkin?
- Throw up after eating?

- Chew large amounts of food, only to spit it out before swallowing?
- Use laxatives, diuretics, or diet drugs to try to control your weight?
- Refuse to miss a day of exercise, even to the exclusion of spending time with others, or even if you're not feeling well?
- Refuse to leave the gym until you have met a certain calorie burn or time goal?
- Exercise early in the morning, late at night, or in the middle of the night, when others are less likely to know what you're doing?
- (If you are female) Have irregular or absent periods?
- Have an intense fear of gaining weight?

Remember that this is not an all-inclusive list; you may have other habits that are just as debilitating. Also, **although saying yes to one or two of these questions doesn't necessarily mean you have a full-blown eating disorder, it could be an indication that there are some areas of concern.** It's important to address those areas to not only help you prevent yourself from developing an eating disorder later, but also feel happier and more satisfied with your life overall.

If you're having trouble convincing yourself that some of your habits are hurting you, check out the following section.

Is what you're doing really "that" big of a deal?

The following list includes some of the dangers associated with disordered behaviors; it is used by permission from CRC Health, via the website http://www.something-fishy.org, one of the most helpful and popular informational websites on eating disorders:

- Malnutrition, Dehydration, and Electrolyte Imbalances
- Edema (swelling of soft tissues due to excess water accumulation)
- Muscular Atrophy
- Impaired Neuromuscular Function
- Paralysis
- Tearing of the Esophagus (due to self-induced vomiting)
- Gastric Rupture
- Gastrointestinal Bleeding
- Esophageal Reflux (sometimes to the point that food cannot be kept down at all)
- Throat/larynx (voice box) cancer (due to acid reflux disorders)
- Insomnia
- Weakness, Fatigue, & Chronic Fatigue Syndrome

- Low Blood Pressure (which can lead to heart arrhythmias, shock, or myocardial infarction; more common in those with anorexia or bulimia)
- Orthostatic Hypotension (sudden blood pressure drop upon sitting/standing; symptoms include dizziness, blurred vision, passing out, heart pounding and headaches)
- High Blood Pressure (more common in those with compulsive overeating or binge eating disorder)
- Low Platelet Count or Thrombocytopenia
- Blood Sugar Level Disruptions (which can indicate liver or kidney problems and can lead to neurological and mental deterioration)
- Diabetes
- Iron Deficiency/Anemia
- Kidney Infection & Failure
- Osteoporosis & Osteopenia
- Degenerative Arthritis
- Dental Problems & Decay; Gum Disease
- Liver Failure
- Poor Circulation, Slowed or Irregular Heartbeat, Arrhythmias, Angina, or Heart Attack
- Amenorrhea (loss of menstrual cycle), Infertility, and/or Polycistic Ovarian Syndrome (PCOS)
- Pregnancy Complications
- Mood Swings and Depression, which can lead to suicide
- Digestive Disturbances (cramps, bloating, constipation, diarrhea, incontinence)
- Peptic Ulcers
- Pancreatitis (when digestive enzymes attack the pancreas; can be caused by vomiting, alcohol consumption, and excessive use of laxatives and diet pills)
- Death due to heart attack/heart failure, lung collapse, internal bleeding, stroke, kidney failure, liver failure, pancreatitis, gastric rupture, perforated ulcer, depression and suicide, or any combination of the above.

Most of these conditions are due to both nutritional deficiencies and the disordered behaviors themselves. I would encourage you to visit the website for more in-depth information about these conditions. Don't fall into the trap of continually telling yourself that it will never happen to you, or that you're "different" somehow from everyone else who has an eating disorder. You're not different, and unless you fix your behaviors, that list is what you have to look forward to.

Despite their consequences, it can be scary to think about living your life without your eating disorder. You have to find new ways to cope with some of your fears and worries, and it takes time before everything starts to feel better. You need to figure out who you really are, and begin to open up and start trusting other people, instead of being afraid they might reject the real you. You have to trust yourself and your abilities, knowing that even if things don't work out exactly like you'd envisioned—they still *will* work out.

Recovery and the process of upcycling are kind of like learning to swim *with* the current of your life, instead of against it. Once you can do that, your life will start clicking into place. Really.

So what comes first? If you haven't already, you need to talk to the people you love about what you're going through. It's not easy, but it's a step that can't be skipped. You need support!

I don't think there's ever an easy way to begin a conversation that includes saying something like, "Oh, by the way, I just threw up those tater tots I ate," or "I think I'm going to go weigh myself and then, based on the number I see, I'm going to decide how much of this food on my plate I need to throw away and how long I need to work out today." For three years, I was determined not to tell a single person about my eating disorder. I thought I could get better on my own, and I didn't want anyone to worry about me. I also didn't really want the accountability that would come from telling.

Still, I felt horrible knowing I was keeping such a huge, horrible secret from the people I cared about most. The longer I continued to bury my secret, the more my anxiety grew, and the worse I felt physically. My muscles were weak and cramped, I was always tired and out of breath, and I had strange tingling sensations in my arms and legs. When I went to sleep at night, my heart would often start to beat a little more quickly, as I thought about the fact that I might very well be slowly killing myself, without anyone I loved having the slightest clue. It was only when I could no longer live with the guilt and anxiety I had from keeping my disorder a secret that I knew I finally had to come clean.

Even though it isn't easy, talking to someone about your eating disorder really is like stepping over the threshold into your recovery: It's how you're going to get the support you need in order to make it through.

There are a few things to keep in mind when getting ready to open up:

Start Talking

No matter what, **don't let anything stop you.** Even though telling my family about my eating disorder isn't on my top-ten list of favorite memories, I knew there was no way I would change unless I did. As long as the problem remained in my head alone, I would always find ways to rationalize it and keep isolating myself from my family, until both my health and my relationships were destroyed.

If possible, **make a plan** about who you're going to talk to first, and how you're going to talk to them. The first person you approach can help you talk to other people. If you're not sure how to begin the conversation, try writing a letter or email first—just make sure you follow up with an in-depth conversation. **If you're not comfortable talking to someone in your family right away (or at all), consider approaching someone else you have a good relationship with**, like a friend, teacher, or clergyperson. Just make sure that person is someone who will take what you are telling them seriously. The last thing you need is a friend who will tell you what you are doing is okay or normal, or that you'll "get over it" in time. You and those you talk to need to be proactive and take the situation seriously.

In my case, I decided to just bite the bullet and tell my mom exactly what was going on. I wasn't exactly sure how she would react (okay, to be perfectly honest I thought she was going to freak out), but I knew I'd have to start talking to her sooner or later. I wanted to get it over with as soon as possible!

The day I first "came out" to my mom about my disorder will remain forever etched in my memory, just as clearly as my first day of kindergarten or my first time behind the wheel (except this time my brother wasn't screaming from the backseat!); it was the mark of one of the hugest educational journeys in my life. It was early in the morning when I first approached her. She had been folding laundry in my father's and her bedroom, and I had just woken up after another night of fragmented, panicked, and guilt-ridden sleep.

I didn't wait for my mother to say good morning before I spoke: "Mom, I have to tell you something…"

"What?" The surprise on my mom's face quickly turned to fear as she saw my own pained expression. She let go of the towel that had been in her hands. "Honey, what's wrong?"

"Mom, I'm...I'm bulimic, Mom."

I remember my mother being quiet for a moment. She didn't "freak out" as I had thought she would. Instead, she just looked at me for a moment. Then, she nodded her head a little and said, "Okay. Okay." She told me that she and my dad had known that something was going on, but that they just didn't know what it was. It was true that a couple of weeks earlier she had taken me to a physician, concerned by some of my eating habits and my change in weight. I had simply told the physician that I had a lot going on in my life. He had then assured my mother that everything they were observing was likely due to stress.

Despite his words of reassurance, my parents' "radar" still seemed to be telling them that something was going on. When I finally told them the truth, they were actually sort of relieved to have an answer. Even though no parent likes to hear that their son or daughter is going through something like an eating disorder, once mine knew what I was dealing with, we could start figuring out *together* what I needed to do to get better.

It's important to **plan to have the conversation at the right time and in the right place.** Don't try to start talking to someone when they're in the middle of a project (I don't think doing laundry counts as a project!) or getting ready for bed, and make sure you're someplace calm and quiet. When you begin talking, **be genuine;** it's the only way you'll be able to help your loved ones understand what you're going through.

No matter what your family is like, you won't always know exactly what their reactions to your news will be like. They may be shocked, or angry, or a number of other things. **Don't take their reactions personally**; you're telling them something pretty big, and they might not know exactly how to respond to it right away. They might also have a lot of misunderstandings and preconceived notions about what you're dealing with. Things will most likely improve as they begin to learn more about what's going on and what they can do to help you. **If you find that you continue to have trouble talking with your family about what you're going through, see if they are willing to go to family counseling with you.** It may also help you to **seek other supportive people to talk to,** like friends, teachers, or church community members.

Let the people in your life know how they can support you, whether that be helping you find a physician, therapist, or dietitian; helping you plan and prepare healthy meals; being available to talk when you're having trouble; or anything else you think you might need. They'll hopefully feel a little more empowered by knowing that there are specific things they can do to help. **Don't place blame on anyone** for your problems—yourself included. Focus on what you can do to get better instead.

Also **ask your loved ones if they have any questions** about what you're going through, and **let them know you'll be open to questions throughout your recovery.** Once my parents saw that I was willing to honestly answer their questions and keep communicating with them about how I was doing, they began to develop a lot more confidence in me and my recovery. In time, I stopped feeling like they were watching everything I ate and did, because we were continually talking about how I was doing. By being more open with them and answering any questions they had, my parents began to trust me again.

Opening up can be scary at first, but it really is the first step towards a much more fulfilling, beautiful, and freer life. These days, my family is amazingly close; I really feel like my family does understand my disorder as well as anyone who's never had one possibly could. Even though they might not have always known exactly what to say, they were *there*, and that's what made all the difference.

If you're still afraid to talk to someone about your disorder, just know that no matter how awkward and uncomfortable things may be in the beginning, they don't have to stay that way. I've learned that the people who are worth my time won't judge me at all. They're actually often able to relate on some level—after all, who doesn't struggle a little with body image, eating habits, insecurity, and emotions? Once you have a bit of support, you'll feel lighter in a way that has nothing to do with weight (Ahh…now doesn't that feel better?)!

Your work doesn't end there. Here's what you do after that first conversation:

The Nuts and Bolts of Recovery

No matter what stage of recovery you're in, **defeat the denial** that always tells you that you don't *really* have a problem, or that what you're doing isn't really even that serious. It doesn't matter how habitual or comfortable some of the things you do have become, or how often you're bombarded by extreme diet and fitness blurbs every time you turn on the television, click your computer mouse, or flip through a magazine. As tough as it may be at first, recovery requires real change.

It took a *really* long time until I could fully confront my own issues. Even after I stopped bingeing and purging, I couldn't let go of some of my unhealthy ideas about food and exercise. I thought I needed to restrict my food and that I needed to exercise every single day for a specific amount of time if I didn't want to get "fat." I thought my fixation on diet and exercise was good, and can you really blame me? The whole world is simply diet-obsessed! Celebrities and bloggers who are obsessive about exercising or following very specific, restrictive diets are praised for being so "devoted" to their health. You may also notice people in your own life who, despite being at perfectly healthy weights, are still always talking about trying to drop a few pounds to look better.

I like to call all of the unhealthy voices and messages around you the "Peanut Gallery." You probably have heard that term being used to refer to people who like to tell you what you should do or think, or how you should spend your time, despite the fact that they don't really know you or what's best for you at all. The members of your own personal Peanut Gallery are people like journalists, celebrities, random strangers, and even negative friends. Nobody in the Peanut Gallery can see what's in your heart. Your job is to **start listening to the voice inside of you that knows the truth.** Are you really going to be happy if you only have that apple for lunch? Is it going to make you feel better if you skip going out with your friends so you can run alone on a treadmill? Does bingeing and purging really get rid of your anxiety? Do you feel relaxed about your food and exercise habits, or does your mind seem consumed with thoughts about food and your body? Even if you're not underweight, are you really as healthy as you could be? (If you're having trouble dealing with some of those questions, rest assured that I'll address them in the following chapters.)

Troy Roness, 23, from North Dakota, said that it's especially important for males with eating or exercise disorders to remember that they are not weak for dealing with what is often considered a "female problem":

> *"...you are stronger than all bodybuilders, professional athletes or any dude on the cover of* Men's Health *magazine. Why? Because you have realized your slips and falls and you are dealing with your internal struggles. Keep acknowledging that you are facing your inner demons and are more than 'man' enough to continue your journey back."*

Do not put recovery off; make the changes *now*. I told myself so many times that I would get better "tomorrow," or when I wasn't so stressed out, or after the holidays when there wasn't so much food around. I told myself that what I was doing was different from what other people were doing—that my habits were "less dangerous" somehow. But the longer I put it off, the more my disorder progressed. In time, I wasn't even able to eat a couple of bites without experiencing so much anxiety that I would inevitably go purge. Even though I thought my eating disorder was giving me a sense of control, it was actually when I had an eating disorder that I had the least amount of control over anything: My brain was so fuzzy from malnourishment that I couldn't focus on any of the things that I really wanted to accomplish. My body became so tired and weak that I stopped doing the things I enjoyed. I stopped really talking to the people I loved, because too much talking means that eventually someone is going to find out what's really going on with you. I was putting both my body and mind at jeopardy, and it continued to get worse until I finally took the first steps to getting better.

In my correspondence with Kelly, 28, from New Jersey, she described how she finally committed to recovery:

> *"It was a big obstacle for me to admit that I needed treatment, that I was worth treatment, and that school was not nearly as important as my health. I ended up leaving school for awhile, and initially I felt guilty, but in the long run I am glad I did. Treatment enabled me to think more clearly, do my work more efficiently, and have the energy to do the work. It was a sacrifice to postpone my education in order to better myself, but when I did graduate, my degree meant so much to me. I had a true appreciation of what I had achieved."*

Even if you don't feel like you have any time to set aside for recovery, it's a necessary investment. You'll be able to accomplish infinitely more after your recovery than you can while you're still struggling with an eating disorder. And better health will also likely give you more time in general.

Schedule the changes you're going to make. Get out your notebook and write down a list of steps to take this week in order to upcycle your life and recover, like finding people to support you and visiting a physician, counselor, and dietitian. Once you've made your list, get out your planner and then actually schedule the days and times when you will complete each task. Also think about who you'd like to have support you, like significant others, parents, friends, or church members. When are you going to talk to them? Schedule a time and then follow through with it. If you're not sure exactly what steps to take, your "team" of support people will be able to help you. The big thing is to make sure you follow your schedule and get those people in your corner as soon as possible!

Upcycle your daily schedule. Take a look at how you spend your time during the day. If you're familiar with Cognitive Behavioral Therapy (something I'll talk more about in Chapter Four), this technique might sound familiar to you: For one week, record everything you do during the day in detail, along with the times when you do them. Make a note of any instances when you struggle more with unhealthy thoughts and behaviors. What time of day was it? What were you doing at that time, and before it?

Show the list to your therapist or counselor, and then with them figure out how you can modify your daily schedule to help you accomplish your goals. How can you upcycle your daily activities? If you spend a lot of time doing something counterproductive to those goals, figure out how you can modify that behavior: If you linger at the table and pick apart your food during meals, make a conscious effort to eat within a certain timeframe by setting a timer or scheduling something to do shortly after your meals. If you feel like bingeing because you get antsy or anxious at certain times, find something to do with your hands, like crocheting, drawing, playing a video game, typing up a story on the computer, or taking a brisk walk (Please keep in mind that if you struggle with over-exercising, you clearly shouldn't be replacing behaviors with more physical activity). Definitely use the "Alternative Activity" list mentioned later on in this chapter when trying to come up with things to do!

An example of a modified daily schedule is on the following page.

Throughout every stage of your recovery, **keep reaching out for support.** Even if you don't feel like you have anyone to talk to, there are plenty of people out there who can help, as long as you just look a little bit. In this book's introduction I mentioned how I began contacting other people in recovery when I was having trouble finding someone to talk to who could relate to what I was going through. Don't ever be afraid to contact people who might be able to help you, whether they're in recovery themselves or you think they might know something about what you're

Upcycled Daily Schedule

Time	Old Activity	New Activity	Resulting Feelings
7:00 a.m.	Get up, run on treadmill.	Get up, walk on treadmill.	Seems okay so far.
8:00 a.m.	Shower	Shower	
9:00 a.m.	Walk to work.	Breakfast, then drive to work.	A little bit uncomfortable.
10:00 a.m.	Arrive at work	Arrive at work	
1:00 p.m.	Eat alone in my car, then take a walk outside.	Meet my friend Lynn for lunch.	Felt a little anxious but was in a better mood at work later.
4:30 p.m.	Nibble on some candy hidden in my desk. Spit half into a napkin to throw away.	Eat an apple with some peanut butter.	Surprised that I actually feel more relaxed. No blood sugar spikes or guilt.
6:00 p.m.	Drive to the grocery store and pick up binge food. Go home and binge/purge.	Drive home and invite my sister over for dinner.	Antsy. Thinking a little bit about bingeing after my sister leaves.
7:30 p.m.	Take a shower.	Spend some time writing in my journal.	I feel more "centered."
8:00 p.m.	Watch TV; hate myself.	Watch one of my favorite TV shows.	Feel fine I guess. Some thoughts of bingeing so I think I'll try to learn to knit to keep my hands occupied.
9:00 p.m.		Read a book.	Good. I hadn't realized how much I missed reading!
10:30 p.m.	Bed	Bed	

going through. You'll probably be amazed by how willing they are to talk!

If you are interested in finding a mentor who has been exactly where you are, you may want to visit the MentorConnect website at http://www.mentorconnect-ed.org/, where people who have recovered are paired up with those in recovery. Although I have not been personally involved in the community as of yet, I do know some wonderful people who have been, and believe that it is worth checking out.

In time, **you'll learn which people in your life are best at helping you in various ways.** These people will make up part of the "team" that will support you throughout your recovery, and beyond. I learned that I could be honest with my dad about slipping up every once in awhile, without him getting upset with me or telling me I was never going to get better. My mom was really encouraging when I needed to talk about some of the "food issues" I had from time to time. Now, post-recovery, my amazing husband (who you'll hear all about later!) is wonderful at showing me how much he loves *me*, no matter how much I weigh or how much I work out.

Make sure you include the right professionals on your "team": You should have a physician who can ensure that you're physically healthy, a counselor or therapist who has been trained to help you understand and manage your emotions, and a dietitian who will be able to help you get your eating back on track. I call these people the "Big Three," because they're integral to your recovery.

Educate your loved ones by giving them information to read, inviting them to come to counseling with you, and continuing to talk to them about what's going on with you. **Make sure you are ready to learn** as well. The world is full of wonderful information and alternative perspectives, but your life will never be enriched if you think you already know everything there is to know about everything. The world is not black and white, and sometimes there are multiple answers to a single question!

Pay attention to what seems to "trigger" your disordered thoughts and feelings: Are there certain things people say that make you want to restrict, binge, purge, etc.? Do you start criticizing your body after watching specific television shows? Are there specific times during the day when you might want to reach for a food you typically binge on?

Once you know your triggers you can figure out how to protect yourself from them and, when that's not possible, how to respond to them in a healthier way. It's one of the most important steps to recovery! See Chapter Two for more on triggers.

Journaling is a wonderful way to help you discover some of your triggers, so **buy yourself a nice journal and some good pens**. Get ready to start paying attention to what's really going on inside you, instead of trying to bury it all away. You can get started by responding to the journal questions at the end of each chapter in this book, or just spending some time free-writing during the day. Journaling will not only help you become more self-aware, but it will also allow you to look back at all of the progress you're making! Chapter Four will have more insight on figuring out your emotions.

Use your support and **trust your support.** You know that little voice that sometimes tells you you're fine and that you can figure everything out on your own? That's not the healthy part of you. The healthy part of you knows you need to stay open with your team and let them help you. **Your healthy self will grow stronger as you begin to nourish your body**: Your emotions will improve, you'll be able to think more clearly, and you'll have more energy. None of this will happen if you're not eating properly (See Chapter Six!).

Heather, 18, from New Hampshire, still recalls her first moments of clarity:

> *"In the early stages of my recovery I was feeling so much happier and free already. I am a cashier at a convenience store, and at work one day, several random people commented on how beautiful my smile was and said I should smile like that more often. Similar comments came from friends, classmates, and teachers in the days to come. Recovery made me feel great in such a way that my happiness radiated out to those around me. I was also amazed by the smiles that I received back. I was so used to being sad and angry at the world, that this was a whole new outlook for me."*

Throughout my own recovery, I began to laugh and smile a lot—something I found very interesting in light of the fact that my ex had once made a comment about how strange it was that I never laughed out loud, even during really funny movies. Once I was out of that relationship and moving past my disorder, I transformed into a much happier, more open person.

Real change doesn't happen overnight, but as long as you're continually taking small steps forward, it does happen. **Make a list of "interventions" to complete:** Interventions are small, healthy lifestyle changes that you add gradually so they're more likely to stick. Even though there are some things you must do immediately, like getting on a healthy meal plan and stopping risky behaviors (such as purging, using diuretics, etc.), you will get overwhelmed if you try to change absolutely everything overnight.

Here are some examples of things to put on your list:

- Stop weighing yourself
- Pick an affirmation to say at every meal
- Eat at an appropriate pace
- Eat dinner with a friend

- Say something nice to yourself every time you're in front of a mirror
- Find one non-physical thing to admire about someone else every day
- (You get the gist—add your own healthy little change here…)
- (…and here…)
- (…and so on!)

Commit to adding one intervention to your life each week. It will only be a matter of time before each of those changes becomes a natural, healthy habit! Pay special attention to areas where you may be struggling, and then come up with more interventions of your own, based on changes you need to make in those areas. Also see Chapter Six for more examples of food-related interventions.

If you're having trouble making changes, **consider recreating your living space.** Doing so can help you shift your perspective a bit, by giving you the sense that you're in a whole new environment (because you are in a new, better life now!). A few years ago I rearranged the furniture in my bedroom to make it easier for me to get to sleep—that way, I wasn't staring at the same things every night and remembering all of the nights when I stayed up anxiously tossing and turning. You can do the same: Put anything out of sight that stirs up uncomfortable feelings, like mirrors, certain pictures, or whatever else you might associate with negative memories. Replace them with art, posters, or inspirational quotes. Your room should be your sanctuary.

Fill your life with positive things. Once you start spending your time doing things you really love, you'll think less about all that negative stuff. You can also **upcycle your responses to negative thoughts and situations by creating an "Alternative Activity" list** with things you can do instead of using food or negative behaviors. Commit to using that list whenever you find yourself in a tough moment.

Your list could look something like this:

Example "Alternative Activity" List

- Finger-paint posters for your room
- Play with paint-by-number books or posters, paint-with-water books, or paper doll books
- Make a collage
- Garden
- Visit a local crafts store and find something new to try
- Play with play-dough; create works of art and then (if you want) destroy them!

- Color pictures of your favorite childhood cartoon characters
- Read a favorite childhood book or another book that will make you feel good
- Curl up with a good puzzle book
- Visit the local library to find a new (or really old!), interesting book
- Write a story you would have liked as a child
- Write in your journal
- Listen to music
- Take a bubble bath
- Put on your jersey and watch a sports game with friends
- Pray
- Do some yoga or tai chi
- Get cozy with your pet
- Play video or computer games, check your e-mail, or browse pro-recovery websites (check out http://www.something-fishy.org/other/websites.php to get started)
- Ride a bike, rollerblade, or skateboard through a park
- Go golfing, shoot some hoops, or fly a kite
- Create a playlist of positive music for your MP3 player
- Take a walk while listening to that positive music
- Get outside and take pictures
- "Camp out" with friends in your living room (think sleeping bags, ghost stories, and flashlights)
- Play board games with your family or friends
- Spend a day shopping to find the best possible item under $10
- Volunteer at an organization you care about
- Visit a local museum or historic site
- Give yourself a manicure/pedicure/facial
- Spend some time playing with your makeup or trying new hairstyles

Laminate the list, print it on a card, or save it on your phone or computer so you'll always have it with you. This list can be a lifesaver!

For a fun spin on the Alternative Activity list, write each of the activities on a separate notecard and then put them in a box. Draw out a notecard when you need an activity to do, and then commit to doing whatever the card says.

To ensure that you always have a ready-to-go response to tough feelings, **make a "fun box"**—a shoebox, bag, or tote filled with items like construction paper, markers, crayons, paints, notebooks, coloring books, scissors, glue, glitter, ribbon, lace, molding clay, puzzle books, comic books, and any other little thing you can get your hands on. Decorate your box, or just keep it plain and discreet. The next time you feel tense, let your creative side take over!

Create a reward system for yourself. If you have spent a lot of money on binge food, diuretics, etc. in the past, put the amount of money you typically spend each week into a savings jar. If you don't typically spend a lot of money on those things, you might want to think about putting money in a jar for every time you don't give in to unhealthy behaviors. Then, periodically reward yourself by spending that money on non-food related things, like new clothes, a day at the spa, or even a weekend trip to somewhere fun. You may want to write what you are planning on buying with the money on the jar, so you have something concrete to focus on anytime you experience a difficult moment.

Stay connected with the people in your life. When your family asks you to go out for dinner or your cousin invites you over for cake on his birthday, even if your first instinct is to stay all curled up in your comfortable little shell at home, *go*—it's when you're in that little shell and away from everyone else that unhealthy behaviors flourish. You miss out on a special kind of joy when you don't have that human connection. It's when I'm with other people, especially the people I care about most, that I feel most alive. The smiles on my nephews' faces when they see me walking in the door make me feel so much happier than staying at home alone with a bowl of cereal, and going out and laughing with my husband and friends on the weekends helps me forget about the little things that are bugging me.

Staying connected also helps you **stay accountable.** Talk regularly with your "team" about how you're doing, even and *especially* when you might not be doing so well. It's crappy to have to tell someone you messed up, but without that support and accountability, you're just putting yourself at the top of a slippery slope again.

Be deliberate and keep trying. Most of the changes you need to make aren't going to just come naturally; for awhile, all those "little" things (like eating a healthy amount, eating the right balance of foods, exercising moderately, not weighing yourself) might feel sort of like learning to brush your teeth with your left hand if you're a rightie: The key is just practicing those changes until they *become* your new habits.

Heather, 36, from Missouri, recovered despite once believing it was impossible:

> *"I really thought I was too far gone. I truly felt that because I had lived more of my life with bulimia than without, I could never get better. I had to believe in myself, and I had to give myself permission to accept help. I have two beautiful kids who need me here. What better reason than that, right? You are* never *too far gone."*

Your life holds an amazing amount of promise, as long as you give yourself the chance to explore that future potential. **Remember that *you* are not your eating disorder.** Author and treatment professional Carolyn Costin was the one who first advised me not to use the term "bulimic" or "anorexic" when talking about someone with an eating disorder. That's because those words are negative labels that shouldn't become part of someone's identity. Rather than saying you are bulimic or anorexic, say instead that you're struggling with bulimia or anorexia. Your eating disorder is separate from you—it's a challenge that you're going to overcome so the *real*, "upcycled" you can start to shine! I'll talk more about how you can start discovering and nurturing your identity in Chapter Three.

Acknowledge your own power. No matter how intense your emotions might get, remember that *you* are still in complete control of your actions. You can choose the path you take from this day forward. Your old, destructive decisions do not have to be the ones you make today. You have a lot to gain from recovery as long as you make the right choice!

Patrick Bergstrom, 26, from Maryland, remembers how he learned that he had to be the center of his own recovery, despite thinking he would be "cured" as soon as he left treatment:

> *"I thought treatment would change my life, and it did. However, treatment is just the beginning toward the road to recovery. Treatment is a safe place to be, and it gives you the tools you need to apply in your everyday life. I was scared when I left the treatment center, but you can't stay there forever. It was tough at first being back in the real world, but my best growth has come from learning out on my own. Treatment is not a cure, but the foundation to a great recovery."*

You have everything in you that it takes to succeed. Above all, **be patient and believe in the process.** You didn't develop an eating disorder overnight, so it won't go away that quickly either. Rachel, 22, from Ontario, Canada described her recovery as a true learning process:

> *"It's not simple. I totally thought recovery would be about going a week or so without skipping meals or throwing up any food. It really, really isn't. I've been surprised by how much recovery is full of surprises. I now understand that there are things ahead of me I still have to learn, that I can't imagine yet. I have had to learn about my emotions. I have had to face the sources of some of my core beliefs about myself. Recovery can't be taught. It can be facilitated—but not even normalizing your eating means you are recovered. It's SO not just about food and weight. The skills that I am learning allow me to deal more adaptively with other people and with life. Recovery really is about getting better: I'm not losing something, but learning how to be myself."*

As long as you're continually and consistently making the changes you need to make, you'll get there. Alicia Houston, 24, from Illinois said that the gifts of recovery are worth every effort:

> *"You know the saying the grass isn't always greener on the other side? Well, in this case it is. You have no idea what is missing in your life until you surrender the power the eating disorder has over you, and reclaim your life. The possibilities will be endless."*

Cheryl Kerrigan, 41, from Massachusetts, and author of *Telling Ed No!*, still remembers the moment she first recognized a transformation in herself:

> *"It was a Tuesday morning and I was at work. I had brought a stack of mail to the postage meter in the back room and began running it through the machine. As I was standing there, a feeling of clarity overcame me. It felt like the blanket that had been covering me up and keeping me in the dark was removed, and all the while the sunlight was hitting my face warming me all over. The air smelled fresh and the sun was warm. As I stood there, the realization that I was thinking more clearly came over me at full-force. I said out loud, 'Oh my God, I can think. I can really concentrate and think.' I was totally amazed. It was like the last piece of a puzzle being put in its place. It was right then that I realized that all the hard work I was doing was paying off. I could feel and identify it for real."*

Even though I had several powerful moments of learning, it wasn't until three years after I considered myself "recovered enough" that I had my own true moment of clarity and understanding, that helped me finally cross over the threshold to true recovery. You'll have to wait until Chapter Eight to find out more about that (or, if we're being honest and you're like me, you might skip ahead and read it right now. It won't have quite the same effect, but I won't get mad).

Next are a few journal questions that will help shape your recovery, followed by a special section for your loved ones, with tips, questions they can ask you, and their own journal questions. At the end of the chapter you'll find a special Q & A section with insight from experts Doris Smeltzer, Carolyn Costin, and Keesha Broome.

Journal Questions

1. What will change throughout my recovery? What will stay the same?

2. What are some concrete goals I have for myself throughout

recovery? What specific steps will I take to reach those goals?

3. What aspects of recovery will be most difficult for me? How can I better prepare myself for those aspects?

Tips for Friends & Family

First, know the signs & symptoms.

If you're reading this book because you suspect your loved one might have an eating disorder, here is a list of signs and symptoms, used by permission from CRC Health, from the Something Fishy website (http://www.something-fishy.org/isf/signssymptoms.php):

Anorexia/Bulimia

1. Dramatic weight loss in a relatively short period of time.
2. Wearing big or baggy clothes or dressing in layers to hide body shape and/or weight loss.
3. Obsession with weight and complaining of weight problems (even if "average" weight or thin).
4. Obsession with calories and fat content of foods.
5. Obsession with continuous exercise.
6. Frequent trips to the bathroom immediately following meals (sometimes accompanied with water running in the bathroom for a long period of time to hide the sound of vomiting).
7. Visible food restriction and self-starvation.
8. Visible bingeing and/or purging.
9. Use or hiding use of diet pills, laxatives, or enemas.
10. Isolation. Fear of eating around and with others.
11. Unusual food rituals such as shifting the food around on the plate to look eaten; cutting food into tiny pieces; making sure the fork avoids contact with the lips (using teeth to scrape food off the

fork or spoon); chewing food and spitting it out, but not swallowing; dropping food into napkin on lap to later throw away.

12. Hiding food in strange places (closets, cabinets, suitcases, under the bed) to avoid eating (Anorexia) or to eat at a later time (Bulimia).

13. Flushing uneaten food down the toilet (can cause sewage problems).

14. Vague or secretive eating patterns.

15. Keeping a "food diary" or list that consists of food and/or behaviors (ie., purging, restricting, calories consumed, exercise, etc.)

16. Preoccupied thoughts of food, weight, and cooking.

17. Visiting websites that promote unhealthy ways to lose weight.

18. Reading books about weight loss and eating disorders.

19. Self-defeating statements after food consumption.

20. Hair loss. Pale or "grey" appearance to the skin.

21. Dizziness and headaches.

22. Frequent sore throats and/or swollen glands.

23. Low self-esteem. Feeling worthless. Often putting themselves down and complaining of being "too stupid" or "too fat" and saying they don't matter. Need for acceptance and approval from others.

24. Complaints of often feeling cold.

25. Low blood pressure.

26. Loss of menstrual cycle.

27. Constipation or incontinence.

28. Bruised or callused knuckles; bloodshot or bleeding in the eyes;

light bruising under the eyes and on the cheeks.

29. Perfectionistic personality.

30. Loss of sexual desire or promiscuous relations.

31. Mood swings. Depression. Fatigue.

32. Insomnia. Poor sleeping habits.

Compulsive Overeating/Binge Eating Disorder

1. Fear of not being able to control eating, and while eating, not being able to stop.

2. Isolation. Fear of eating around and with others.

3. Chronic dieting on a variety of popular diet plans.

4. Holding the belief that life will be better if they can lose weight.

5. Hiding food in strange places (closets, cabinets, suitcases, under the bed) to eat at a later time.

6. Vague or secretive eating patterns.

7. Self-defeating statements after food consumption.

8. Blames failure in social and professional community on weight.

9. Holding the belief that food is their only friend.

10. Frequently out of breath after relatively light activities.

11. Excessive sweating and shortness of breath.

12. High blood pressure and/or cholesterol.

13. Leg and joint pain.

14. Weight gain.

15. Decreased mobility due to weight gain.

16. Loss of sexual desire or promiscuous relations.

17. Mood swings. Depression. Fatigue.

18. Insomnia. Poor Sleeping Habits.

Please remember that many people with eating disorders may not fit into a specific category: There may be weeks or months when they are very restrictive with their eating, and other times when they eat large amounts of food (with or without purging.) Others may seem to have relatively normal eating habits, but remain overly (and negatively) fixated on what they are eating and/or the appearance of their bodies. Some less commonly-recognized eating disturbances are orthorexia—a fixation on food that is considered "pure" and healthy, and body dysmorphic disorder—excessive negative concern over a perceived flaw (or flaws) in one's body.

Also remember that just because someone isn't underweight, it doesn't mean they don't have an eating disorder. People suffering with these illnesses can be anywhere on the weight continuum, from extremely thin to extremely overweight. If you have a "feeling" that something might be going on, follow your instincts. It's better to be safe!

It's not about food. Really.

No matter how great that cheeseburger tastes and smells, eating it is not going to magically make any of your loved ones' problems go away. Eating disorders are complex, and each person's reasons for developing one are different. Many people with eating disorders feel a sense of control over food and their body, even if they feel like they can't control anything else in their lives. Disordered behaviors can also be a way for someone to try to cope with or avoid difficult emotions. People who develop eating disorders are often (but not always) those who have trouble expressing their feelings to others: For example, if someone with an eating disorder gets upset with a parent or spouse, they may deal with their frustration by bingeing and purging, instead of approaching their loved one to discuss the issue. Thanks to our thin-obsessed society, eating disorders are also more likely to affect those with poor self-esteem, who may equate their ability to stay thin with their self-worth.

Reading the rest of this book should help you better understand some of the things your loved one is going through, as well as how you can help them.

Don't forget the basics.

Encourage your loved one to put in place the "Big Three" by helping them find a physician, counselor or therapist, and dietitian who have experience working with people with eating disorders.

Don't try to "fix" me yourself.

No matter what you do or say, it's ultimately up to your loved one to do what he or she needs to do in order to get better.

Educate yourself.

There are a lot of misconceptions out there about eating disorders; it will be easier for your loved one to talk to you if they feel like you really understand what they're going through.

Ask questions.

There's no better way to try to understand your loved one's situation than to actually ask them about it. Try to ask questions at a time when your loved one is more likely to be relaxed. Immediately before, during, and after mealtimes are usually not the best times to be asking questions unless you're asking what you can do to support them.

See the family section within each chapter for specific questions to ask your loved one!

Listen.

The better you become at it, the better your loved one will become at opening up to you.

Just be there.

Your simple presence may be a huge comfort. Traci, 37, from California suggested that you stay connected with your loved one, even if they seem to be pushing you away or isolating themselves. She noted, "They very much want your love and support; they're just so lost in the sickness that they don't know how to love themselves, let alone let others love them."

Don't blame yourself.

Eating disorders are complex, and you may not ever know exactly what combination of things brought on your loved one's struggles. My sister has the same genetics as me and was raised in the same family—but she has never had any eating or exercise disorder. Remember: No one ever wins in the blame game!

Remember that there is no single "cure."

Just as there is no one specific cause, there is no single cure: It may take some trial-and-error before your loved one figures out what kind of treatment plan works best for them. The key is to always give each plan a consistent, honest effort.

Questions Friends & Family Should Ask

1. What would you like me to know about what you're dealing with?
2. What are your goals for your recovery? What are the biggest challenges you think you'll face?
3. What can I do to support you?

Journal Questions for Friends & Family

1. What questions do I have about eating disorders and recovery, and where will I go to find answers (beyond what's in this book)?
2. What are my concerns about some of the specific things my loved one is going through?
3. How can I be supportive?

Q & A with Doris Smeltzer

Doris Smeltzer left her teaching position when her 19-year-old daughter Andrea died after one year of bulimic behaviors. She has since devoted her life to eating disorder prevention through the Andrea's Voice Foundation non-profit she co-founded with her husband. Doris holds a master's degree in counseling psychology and is the author of Andrea's Voice: Silenced by Bulimia*; Gurze Books' "Advice for Parents" blog; and co-author of Chapter 21 in* Treatment of Eating Disorders: Bridging the Research-Practice Gap. *Doris is developing a family and friends support group curriculum for the eating disorder field based on her Internet radio show, "Savor Yourself."*

Q: I have an eating disorder but nobody knows about it. How do I tell my friends and family what's going on?

A: The fact that you are ready to talk about the eating disorder (ED) is HUGE! I would want to attempt to ensure that whomever you reach out to first is a person whom you feel can hear what you have to say with compassion and without judgment. That person may be a family member or friend...or not. In that case, maybe a trusted teacher, a minister, a school counselor, a good neighbor. You want to be sure that you make an appointment with the person and that you find a time and place where you can have some privacy when neither of you are in a hurry or under a lot of pressure (such as right before an exam, before a big holiday event, etc.).

If you find that the words do not come, bring a handout on the topic (the National Eating Disorders Association (NEDA) has some great one-page sheets on their website at http://bit.ly/WNDpSs or you can find links on our Andrea's Voice Foundation web site at http://bit.ly/S7vVOp) and our Foundation (email: doris@andreasvoice.org) is always willing to send out as many brochures as needed, free of charge. Ask your confidant to read the handout/brochure and then tell them that is what you are struggling with (this idea is adapted from a story from Jenni Schaefer, who often tells of hiding a brochure for her boyfriend to find when she found it difficult to say the words).

If sharing with your family still seems too difficult you could ask this trusted person to come with you to support you while you inform them of your struggles.

If for some reason the first few people you choose to talk to do not take what you say seriously, or deny that you have a problem, please do not be discouraged. Sadly, these are not uncommon reactions…you need to keep sharing until you find someone who takes your words and your illness seriously so that you can work together to come up with a plan for treatment.

Q: I just told my family about my eating disorder and they didn't react well. What's going on with them?

A: I know that as a parent it is so very difficult for us to hear that our child is suffering from a serious illness—we truly want to resist hearing this information with every fiber of our being because we fear the death of our child. Revealing an eating disorder is confounded by the fact that these illnesses carry with them a tremendous amount of stigma and shame, due to misunderstandings, misconceptions, and misinformation. A parent may think: If my child suffers in this way what does that say about me as a mother (or father, step-parent, guardian)?

The culture speaks "anorexic" ("these foods are bad, those are good," "thin is healthy, fat is not," "no pain, no gain," etc.) and the media tells us that ultra-thin for females and six-pack abs for males are the only acceptable body shapes. It may be, too, that family members struggle with their own "disordered" eating behaviors and "distorted" thoughts around body, food, and weight. This often limits our ability to see eating disorder struggles as abnormal or dangerous.

Please remember that anger is often a secondary emotion. Our primary emotion may be guilt or fear…these emotions are more difficult for us to admit. Anger is direct, quick, and can often get us off the hook so that we do not have to look at our more difficult-to-express feelings. All of this to say, family is not perfect. We're going to react in unhelpful or inappropriate ways more times than we'd ever like to admit. And we certainly cannot ask a child to maintain a level of emotional maturity that we as a parent cannot muster…especially a child who is ill. Sometimes the best way to respond is to request a postponement and return to the subject when feelings are less intense. Obviously, if the reactions never soften, please see my responses to the previous question about finding someone who *can* hear what you need to say and can provide needed support during your healing journey.

Q: What do I need to know about how my family and friends are feeling throughout my recovery? What should I do and say to help them?

A: This is a tough question...because what we feel about your struggle may be predicated on our understanding of why you are struggling. As you know, eating disorders are difficult to comprehend. If I am stuck in my erroneous thoughts that this is a choice you've made and/or a vie for attention, then your struggles make even less sense to me and sadly, you may pay a great emotional price for my misunderstanding.

I would like to believe, though, that most of us, as parents, ache deeply when our children struggle or are in pain. We also live continually with the fear that we could lose you to this disease. Sometimes, we have to deny the severity of your illness just to allow us to get through the day. Please understand that for the vast majority of us: No matter how we act or what we say, the thought of living our lives without *you* hurts at a cellular level. The glimpses of how we would feel without you here can rob us of our sanity and may even throw us into a state of suspended animation. Just as we need to be patient with you and your process of healing, please be patient with us and our attempts at supporting you in your recovery.

Andrea kept assuring me that the eating disorder was not my fault…I now realize how much of her energy was expended on reassuring me. The sadness is that this is an illness of disconnections—not only do you disconnect from yourself, but the eating disorder often requires that you disconnect from nearly everyone else as well. So the situation is one where what is desperately needed is for all of us to remain connected…yet that can be the most difficult thing to achieve. I think I would want for Andrea to be honest with me, sharing her truths "without judgment" as Carolyn Costin would say. And that I, too, could speak my truths to her without judgment—with both of us being willing to work at repairing the connection when/if we miss the mark.

Q: What else should I keep in mind about my family?

A: Although I mentioned this briefly in another response, I think it is paramount for families to get into counseling together. Finding a therapist with expertise and experience with eating disorders is preferable (they're more likely to understand the unique triggers and challenges of the illness) but if not, finding someone who comes highly recommended is the next best thing. Not only will we be learning (or being reminded of) valuable relationship-building skills, but we can receive guidance on how to minimize triggers in our home so that it is an environment supportive of healing. Family therapy will definitely allow us to relate to or understand our loved ones and their feelings throughout recovery. As unbelievable as it may seem, this experience has the potential to become a valuable journey of self-discovery for all involved.

Q: What kinds of things can my loved ones help me with throughout my recovery, and what should be left up to the professionals?

A: Whether we are intimately involved in the treatment process (i.e. following a protocol for Family-Based Treatment (FBT; http://bit.ly/10VMEHa) or are relying on a treatment team for re-feeding, etc., we need to understand and feel confident in the role we play in the healing process. The specific things that come under the purview of the family versus the professionals will depend on which treatment path is chosen. Some of the things family members can do, no matter which protocol is followed, include: Loving and supporting our child while setting clear and consistent boundaries that allow all of us to feel respected, loved, and not judged, getting ourselves into therapy (hopefully for the entire family) so that we can work through our reactions and (re)learn helpful communication skills and boundary-setting, reading books and websites, going to conferences, talking to experts, following guidelines set by the treatment protocol, attending support groups for families online or in our communities, and modeling self-love and appropriate self-care.

Q & A with Carolyn Costin, MFT, M.A., M.ED., and Keesha Broome, M.A., MFT

Carolyn Costin is an author, therapist, and specialist in the field of eating disorders. She is known for her activism and advocacy and for her long-held view that those with eating disorders can become fully recovered. Carolyn has herself been recovered from anorexia for over 30 years. She is the founder and executive director of The Eating Disorder Center of California, and Monte Nido Eating Disorder Treatment Center and its affiliates. Carolyn's books, Your Dieting Daughter, The Eating Disorder Source Book, 100 Questions and Answers about Eating Disorders, *and* 8 Keys to Recovery from an Eating Disorder, *are popular with professionals, sufferers, and families of those who are suffering. Aside from running her eating disorder clinics and writing, Carolyn educates and trains professionals on eating disorder awareness, prevention, and treatment through lectures and workshops at organizations, schools, and groups throughout the United States, and at both national and international conferences. A former Board Trustee of the National Eating Disorder Association (NEDA), Carolyn currently serves on the board of the International Association of Eating Disorder Professionals (IAEDP). Carolyn is a fellow of the Academy of Eating Disorders (AED) and a member of the National Association of Anorexia Nervosa and Associated Disorders (ANAD), the Eating Disorder Coalition (EDC), the American Association of Marriage and Family Therapists (AAMFT), and serves on the editorial board for* Eating Disorders: The Journal of Treatment and Prevention.

Keesha Broome is a licensed marriage and family therapist specializing in the treatment of eating disorders. After recovering from anorexia and exercise addiction, she received her Master's degree in clinical psychology from Pepperdine University. She is the Assistant Clinical Director of the Monte Nido Treatment Center, one of Carolyn Costin's residential programs, and also sees clients in an outpatient setting. Before coming to the field of psychology, she worked as a journalist in New York City and Texas. Keesha still pursues her passion for the written word through various writing projects, including a blog on the Gurze website. She is committed to the prevention and treatment of eating disorders and related issues through writing, speaking, and her work at Monte Nido.

Q: Where Do I Begin in Recovery?

A: Eating disorders are serious illnesses that can cause serious medical complications. Because of these possible complications, it is important to seek medical attention. If possible, find a physician who has some knowledge of eating disorders. Before scheduling an appointment, ask the physician if they have experience working with eating disorders and how extensive their knowledge is. If you are having trouble finding a knowledgeable physician, ask your therapist for his/her recommendations (more on finding a therapist below).

Have your physician take blood work, do an EKG (a test that measures electrical activity in the heart), and do a bone scan to measure bone density.

Once you have seen a physician, the next important step is to find a therapist. If at all possible, it is critical to find a therapist who has training and experience in the treatment of eating disorders. There are many internet resources to help you find one. A few helpful sites for finding a therapist in your area are:

Eating Disorder Referral and Information Center:	http://www.edreferral.com
Something Fishy Website on Eating Disorders:	http://www.something-fishy.org
International Association of Eating Disorder Professionals:	http://www.iaedp.com
Academy for Eating Disorders:	http://www.aedweb.org
Gurze Books:	http://www.bulimia.com

A dietitian is another significant part of your treatment team. The sites listed above also have names of dietitians or your therapist might have someone he/she works with specifically. Getting your team in place is one of the foundational pieces for healing.

Q: What are the different types of treatment/treatment program options?

A: There are several options for treatment depending on your needs, symptoms, and insurance coverage. Here are the basic levels of care:

Inpatient: This is the most acute level of care and most often takes place in a hospital setting. Inpatient treatment is needed if someone is medically compromised or if their symptoms pose an immediate risk. Medical supervision is the main concern at this level of care and often therapy takes a backseat to this goal.

Residential: One step down from inpatient, this level of care is also 24 hours a day but takes place in a residential setting. It may or may not include 24-hour nursing care but requires that the person is medically stable (meaning no immediate risk). Residential treatment includes psychotherapy and nutrition therapy and often many other kinds of treatment modalities. Residential programs are especially helpful in treating eating disorders because they provide containment around the behaviors while also addressing the psychological component and fostering insight. Furthermore, residential settings allow for necessary exposure to help overcome issues with food, weight, and body image that are unlikely in an inpatient setting, For example, clients have the opportunity to slowly practice and integrate recovery behaviors such as shopping, cooking, and exercise. Clients have the ability to take ownership of making appropriate choices while still being monitored day and night.

Partial Hospitalization Program (PHP): This is a partial hospital program or Day Treatment. It generally involves five to six days of programming a week for most of the day. Clients in day treatment do not live at the facility so there is more freedom and less structure on nights and weekends. This level of treatment can be successful for motivated individuals and those who have sufficient support outside of program hours. Some people step down to day treatment after an inpatient or residential stay. Day treatment is often tried in order to prevent admission to a 24-hour setting.

Intensive Outpatient Program (IOP): This type of treatment typically involves a few evenings a week of group therapy and often a structured meal. Clients may be working or in school during the day and then attending the program on the designated evenings. People need to be motivated and in appropriate physical condition to attend.

Outpatient Therapy: There are a variety of outpatient therapies. "Outpatient" means seeing a professional in that person's private practice office on a predetermined schedule. Your outpatient treatment team may include a therapist, dietitian, and psychiatrist. You may pay for these services out of pocket, or if you have insurance your plan may pay for a specific number of sessions per calendar year or some other option.

The level of care you choose should be based on your specific needs as well as what is feasible for your life. While one person might need acute care due to medical risk factors, another person might find that they are making progress in outpatient therapy. Some people find the structure of an IOP or day treatment to be more appropriate. Sometimes, individuals start in one level of care and then realize they need more support and transfer to a higher level of care. If you feel that outpatient therapy is not enough, enlist your outpatient team to help you determine what is best for you.

Within these levels of care, there are different kinds of treatment. Some programs utilize the 12-step model (like that used by programs such as Alcoholics Anonymous) while others do not believe that eating disorders are addictions and thus they are treated differently. For example, in the addiction community the belief is that recovery is an ongoing process taken one day at a time; but at our treatment centers, the philosophy is that you can fully recover from an eating disorder. There is actually a growing body of research that validates this belief. Various studies have shown that although it takes time, people can completely heal from their eating disorders: Their behaviors become a thing of the past, and not something fought against one day at a time. There is also research showing that working with staff who have recovered themselves can be helpful in the recovery process.

If you have insurance, contact them to find out what treatment options are available to you. You can get a list of programs from them and then do your own research on the internet. As stated previously, a good place to start searching for treatment programs is http://www.edreferral.com.

Q: What advice do you have for those who are having trouble getting insurance coverage and paying for treatment?

A: Dealing with insurance can be a daunting and frustrating task. When looking for an insurance policy, remember that you are the consumer and should get what you're paying for. There are some basic guidelines to look for when shopping around for the right policy. Make sure that "parity" applies to the policy. Parity means that any mental health diagnosis must be treated in the same way by insurance as any medical diagnosis would be. In many states anorexia and bulimia are parity diagnoses, but several states have not included these diagnoses yet.

If your state has parity for anorexia and bulimia your treatment is not supposed to be subjected to a time limit; therefore, as long as you meet the medical necessity of treatment for an eating disorder, you should be allowed treatment at the appropriate level of care. Parity is definitely great progress for the mental health field, but it does not guarantee that care will be covered. Insurance companies so far have been able to determine their own criteria for medical necessity. Unfortunately, this means that they can deny coverage based on their definition. The American Psychiatric Association does have guidelines to help dictate, and we often cite these when discussing medical necessity with an insurance company.

Make sure that your insurance policy has residential benefits. The bottom line is that you want a policy that covers the most for the longest time to ensure that you get the care that you need.

If you have difficulty with your insurance coverage, know that you have rights. Be your own advocate. Stand up for yourself. Contact your insurance and ask for a case manager so that you can discuss your case and ask for what you need. If your insurance company is unwilling or unable to help you, you also have a right to file a complaint or to go outside of the company. You can contact the Department of Managed Health or Department of Insurance for your state and ask for an independent medical review. If you continue to have difficulty getting the care that you need or if an egregious decision is made, you have the right to hire an attorney to help you dispute your case. Go to the National Eating Disorders Association website at http://www.nationaleatingdisorders.org/insurance-resources for more information on how to fight back and advocate for your rights.

Outside of insurance coverage and paying out-of-pocket for treatment, there seem to be limited options for finding treatment funding. You may want to explore possible aids or grants available through your school, community, or religious resources.

2 So You Dropped Your Fork: Defeating challenges & roadblocks

"To accomplish great things, we must not only act, but also dream; not only plan, but also believe."

– *Anatole France*

The day before I told my parents I had bulimia, my mom brought home about six partial cakes of all different flavors, all topped and decorated with my favorite powdered sugar icing. As a Family and Consumer Sciences teacher, she sometimes had extra food to bring home after some of her cooking classes. When I saw all those cakes, I was in heaven and hell at the same time. I wanted so badly to just be able to stop bingeing and purging, but it seemed like every time I made up my mind to do it, something would weaken my resolve.

All that cake was a "trigger" for me—it sort of flipped the invisible switch inside me that made me want very badly to engage in unhealthy behaviors. I love cake, but had told myself so many times that I "couldn't" have it, that it felt nearly impossible for me to ever have just one piece. I also hated seeing so much food sitting around and knowing it might go to waste if I didn't eat it. My cravings would go crazy after a couple of bites; I'd eat way more than I felt comfortable with, and then the fear and shame would set in. I'd purge. I'd feel a little bit better, and then a whole lot worse. My head would spin and I'd tell myself that it had been the last time. I would be stronger than my cravings next time. I didn't need anyone else to help me. I could do it on my own.

And then, I'd walk back into the kitchen and see six cakes, of all different flavors, and topped with my favorite powdered sugar icing.

The morning after my mom brought the cakes home was the day I cornered her in her bedroom and told her the truth about my eating disorder. I couldn't get better on my own, not only because I needed emotional support, but also because I needed my family to understand what they could do to help make our home a healthy environment for me. We had to learn together about what helped and hindered my recovery. My mom wrapped up the cake and stuck it in our freezer, out of sight. She continued to do the same thing whenever she brought home extra food later. Once you start understanding your own triggers, you can talk to the supportive people in your life about how they can help you overcome them.

Here's how to get started:

Upcycle Your Responses to Triggers

Practice awareness. Besides seeing multiple cakes or other goodies, some of the things that triggered me were eating food that wasn't on my meal plan, having too much unstructured time, not getting enough sleep, hearing people talk about dieting, and emotions like anxiety or sadness. Pay attention when you start to have negative feelings, and write down what was going on right before you had them: Did someone say something to you that upset you? Did you see an image in a magazine that bothered you? Are you tired?

Once you know what your triggers are, do your best to immunize yourself from them. Don't spend time with people who bring you down. Tell your family and friends if it bothers you when they talk about dieting, weight loss, or any other topics. Don't read magazines that always have skinny models or advertisements for diet drugs. Set an early bedtime for yourself, and schedule a quick nap if you need to. **Schedule activities to take place during times when you normally binge, purge, over-exercise, etc.** I know it might seem obvious, but you need to actually make a specific plan for protecting yourself in the first place. Set boundaries, and stick to them!

"Upcycle" your responses to triggers by having a plan ready for those times when you can't prevent them. You're not always going to be able to control what you see or hear. When I hear people who are perfectly normal in size talking about skipping meals to drop some weight, I might question the three healthy meals I've eaten throughout the day. That doesn't mean I'm going to stop eating. Instead, I'll try to reframe my thoughts, take a quick walk to clear my head, or talk about it with someone in my family. They're always great at helping me put things in perspective again and remember how tired and cranky I always felt before I started eating healthy.

When something flips your switch and makes you want to go back to old habits, do something positive instead: Talk to someone about how you're feeling, and start going through your "Alternative Activity" list (See Chapter One if you haven't yet) until you feel better. Alicia Houston, 24, from Illinois, said she used to write out Bible verses on cards to memorize or meditate on if she began to feel triggered around mealtimes. Paint a picture, play some frisbee golf, dance to your favorite music, write a story, organize your closet, or play with your cat. If you're at work or school, start checking things off of your to-do list.

Hilary Crist, 27, from California, made her own personal "emergency list" with four steps that she methodically follows. She said the list provides "the chance to first try to get through the moment on my own, which is what I am more comfortable with, but also gives me a structure to follow so that if I try to do things on my own and need additional help, reaching out is an option."

Here is Hilary's list:

1. **Opposite to Emotion.** First, Hilary will do the opposite of whatever negative behavior she feels like doing. Once she's done that, if she is still struggling, she goes on to Number Two.

2. **Go to Your Own Space—Deep Breathing and/or Meditation.** Hilary's space is upstairs, away from the kitchen and any bathrooms. It is a room that she turned into a relaxing space that is free of distractions. She keeps her recovery materials and books there, including a meditation book with positive thoughts that has been helpful to her.

3. **Make a "Pros and Cons" List.** If Hilary is still caught up in negative thoughts she writes a list of the pros and cons of engaging in eating disorder behaviors. She said that because the cons always outweigh the pros, looking at the list helps her engage her "more rational side of the mind." Her list helps her recognize that bingeing and purging will make her feel worse, without solving any of her problems.

4. **Call Someone Supportive.** If none of the above steps work, Hilary calls someone she can talk to, like her boyfriend, therapist, or friends who have recovered from eating disorders themselves.

Hilary said she feels empowered by having a plan of attack, so she can make positive choices instead of resorting to disordered behaviors. She added that her list is a very personal list of the things that work for her, and that what is helpful for her may not be for someone else.

Go ahead and try Hilary's list if you think it might help you, or feel free to come up with a list of your own. Beyond that, there are some other things you can do to make yourself feel more at ease in an uncomfortable moment. First, **ground yourself,** and **be present.** When your mind starts to go in a million different directions, stop for a minute and look around. Pay attention to all of the little details in your surroundings, like the textures of the carpet below you and the ceiling above. If there are people around you, get actively involved in their conversation. Get out of your head and back into the world.

Listen to your healthy voice. If you've read Jenni Schaefer's book *Life Without Ed*, you're familiar with this concept. In the book, Jenni talks about separating your healthy thoughts from your unhealthy thoughts, by attributing the unhealthy thoughts to your eating disorder. She refers to her unhealthy thoughts as being the voice of "Ed" (a name derived from the initials for eating disorder) and looks at the process of her recovery as being like getting a divorce from someone who is destructive to her.

Throughout my life, and especially through my recovery, I've been very aware of the fact that I often have conflicting thoughts: Should I act on impulse, or should I do what I know is right—even if what's "right" seems more difficult? Should I listen to the disordered thoughts that tell me to skip lunch or binge on junk food, or should I eat the balanced meal I've planned, even if that's not what I feel so compelled to do in the moment?

If you're a religious person like me, you may also choose to recognize your healthy thoughts as being spiritual guidance, to help you stay on the path that will help you live the kind of life you desire. Unhealthy thoughts are deterrents to that guidance.

On another level, stay aware of all of the influences that are around you, like your family, friends, and the media. Certain relatives may have some unhealthy eating habits that affect you when you're at home or at family get-togethers. Some of your friends may talk critically about others' bodies. Images you see on television, in magazines, or online may glorify unhealthy and even unreal body types. With all of these influences around you, it's absolutely essential that you work to keep your *own* voice at the center of everything: How will *you* choose to eat? What's *your* body supposed to look like? How are you going to keep your body as healthy as possible?

Counter your negative thoughts with the rational truth, and remember that **it is your choice to respond to your triggers in a healthy way.** If you'd like, take the advice of April, 16, from Idaho, and **write a letter to your eating disorder** that says why you deserve to eat and be happy and healthy. April said that rereading her letter often helped her calm down in difficult moments.

As long as you continue to make the right choices, it will only be a matter of time before all your triggers won't bother you so much anymore. Now when I go visit family over the holidays and see about twelve new kinds of goodies to try, I know I don't have to try everything at once; it will still be there later on or the next day if I want some. See Chapter Seven for some tips on managing holiday eating and other specific challenging eating situations.

You may not always respond to your triggers in the most positive way. After all, you are human and habits are incredibly hard to change. However, you *are* capable of making the right choices. Any lapse you may experience does not have to mean a full-blown *relapse.*

Here's what you can do to get back on track after a slip:

Defeat Lapses

Figure out what happened, and then figure out what you're going to do if it happens again. What triggered you? Was it a comment, a specific situation, or a certain type of food?

Why did it trigger you? Are you feeling stressed out or upset about something? Are you tired or overwhelmed? What's *really* going on?

Create a "Red Flags" list. As suggested by Carolyn Costin in the Q & A section later on in this chapter, make a list of behaviors that may indicate you are struggling or experiencing a lapse in your recovery, like exercising alone in your bedroom at night, talking about weight or body fat, or reading the food labels of everything you eat. If you're having trouble thinking of things, refer to the "How do I know if some of my behaviors are disordered?" checklist in Chapter One. Show the list to your loved ones, therapist, and dietitian, so they can help you stay accountable and recognize when you might need a little bit of extra support. This list can keep you from getting too far off track if you ever do begin to slip a little.

Stay accountable and stay in touch with those who are supporting you, even and especially if you have a setback. They'll help you figure out what you can do to prevent it from happening again in the future. **Don't beat yourself up about your mistakes;** after all, no one is perfect. However, **don't let a slipup (or several) turn into an excuse to go back to old habits.** Look at the big picture and remind yourself what it is you are trying to accomplish: **What actions are going to help you achieve your goals in the long run?**

Also **be mindful that you're not substituting new unhealthy behaviors for some of your old behaviors**. You're still off track if you find yourself continually coming up with reasons for never eating certain foods or entire food groups (Chapter Seven has some tips for reincorporating challenging foods). Even if you feel like you're improving because you aren't bingeing and purging anymore, you're still not where you need to be if you're now restricting food, working out after every single meal, or chewing and spitting out food without swallowing it. In regards to the last issue—chewing and spitting—even if it seems like a "harmless" way to hold on to disordered behaviors, engaging in it will make it nearly impossible for you to be able to manage food cravings and control your eating habits.

Don't cheat yourself out of a full recovery. It isn't easy, but I am a strong advocate that it is possible. Let me repeat that, except in big letters:

It is possible to *fully* recover!

As you'll see in the following chapters, my own life is dramatically different today than it was a few years ago, and it's all because I made all of the changes I'll share with you in this book. When I went to college in the midst of my eating disorder I was shy, insecure, afraid, and depressed. These days, even though I'm still a little soft-spoken at times, it's easy for me to talk to people because I feel good about myself. I still worry about some things more than I need to, but I don't usually lose sleep over it. And the best thing? I'm *genuinely* happy. There will always be bumps in life, but I have a completely different attitude than what I had before. I know I'm tough (and persistent) enough to get through my challenges now.

I'm just one of many who believe in the possibility of 100% recovery. Alethia, 26, from Arizona said it just takes awhile for you to be able to "undo" the distorted ideas and negative behaviors that you've learned over time:

> *"I have met many, and am now one, who is fully recovered. It is possible and it can happen. It takes time; it took a long time to be as sick as I was, and it took even longer to undo all the injustice I had done to my mind. Just because recovery may take a month, a year, a few years, it doesn't mean that it isn't there to be had. The damage we do to our minds and all the learned behaviors and underlying negative thoughts we tell ourselves without even thinking about it—it takes time to retrain yourself and your mind, but it is doable. Even as overwhelming as an eating disorder feels and as impossible as it feels to recover, it isn't. You weren't created with an eating disorder even if it started at a very young age...it was learned, it was created over time to cope, and you can unlearn it and cope in new ways. You are NOT your eating disorder. You may struggle with one but it is not who you are."*

Jody Lanham, 55, from Ohio, said that her whole view of herself has changed as a result of recovery:

> *"There were many thoughts I had in the early months (of recovery)—fear of relapse, fear of weight gain, fear of not learning to love myself and become a person who is valuable and intelligent and caring and kind—fear that I would never feel like the person I hoped to become once I 'recovered.' Recovery is a process and I can see how it has evolved, how I feel new feelings and discover new abilities, and allow myself to face new challenges. It has been three years for me now, and in all honesty, I don't feel like someone who is in recovery or who 'had' an eating disorder. I feel like a 'normal' person who does things, goes places, talks to people and eats meals, without all the troubling thoughts and considerations and excuses and doubts that*

accompanied all that and more when I was ill."

I was also one who used to subscribe to the notion that you couldn't fully recover; however, those were the days when I didn't *want* to let go of all of my little habits. I held onto behaviors because they were like a security blanket to me. It's more comfortable to stay stuck in a rut; the problem is, you never get anywhere. As long as you stay stuck, your mind will never be fully in your life or on your goals. Time keeps passing, but nothing gets better for you. **Be honest with yourself about all of your habits and what effects they may be having on you.** Are you really happy staying right where you are?

Here are a few examples of things that will keep you stuck; I like to call them "Recovery Roadblocks":

Remove Your Roadblocks

- Eating the same things all the time
- Eating foods solely based on their calorie counts
- Avoiding specific foods or food groups
- Eating only at certain times during the day
- Paying obsessive attention to each and every little thing you put in your mouth
- Hiding portions of food under your plate or in your napkin
- Intentionally under-eating, even slightly
- Maintaining a rigid exercise schedule, without regular rest days
- Continuing to compare your body to other people's bodies
- Fixating on the shape or size of certain parts of your body
- Weighing yourself
- Not allowing yourself time to relax during the day
- Hiding any of your habits from others because you know they'd question them

Go back and read that last one again: If you have a feeling that someone might think one (or more) of your behaviors aren't quite "right," you need to listen to that feeling.

If you notice any of these roadblocks (or others) in your life, talk to those who are supporting you about why you're experiencing them, and how you can overcome them. Are you still harboring some of those fears that kept you in your eating disorder? Are you afraid to push past the barriers that are keeping you from reaching a full recovery? No matter how far along you are, don't let yourself get complacent about some of your behaviors; stay mindful of your actions and the reasons behind them, so you can recognize when you might be slipping backward a little.

Devise effective counter-thoughts and actions. For each of your roadblocks, pay attention to how some of your thoughts may be influencing your behavior in those areas (Chapter Four will have additional information on how your thought patterns affect you): For example, if you're having trouble incorporating variety in your meal plan, you may find that you've been telling yourself you can't change your way of eating because you'll gain weight. If this is the case, you can upcycle that thought by replacing it with something more positive, like, "My body cannot be fully nourished with a narrow, limited, or rigid food list." Then, with your therapist, dietitian, or someone else whose opinion you respect, come up with a plan for how you can upcycle your behaviors. You may decide to add one new food each day, or try new versions of the foods you are currently eating. Substitute bread, pretzels, crackers, or popcorn for the rice cakes you normally snack on, try a different kind of fruit or vegetable with your lunch, or even start with different brands or flavors of some of your usual choices.

How about cherries instead of your apple-a-day? How about walnuts instead of almonds? Why not try asparagus or squash instead of just broccoli? Or, if you're one of those people who are *really* stuck in their routine, how about just switching the *order* in which you eat some of your food for a day or two first? How about steaming your carrots instead of just eating them raw?

If your roadblock is exercising more than you should, because you find yourself thinking something like, "I am going to get out of shape if I work out less," you can upcycle that thought by saying, "I only need to exercise a moderate amount in order to stay healthy and stay in shape. If I work out excessively, I'm actually going to be in worse shape and feel worse physically." You can then choose to upcycle your behavior by going to the gym with a friend, or scheduling appointments to occur within a reasonable amount of time after your workout (Check out Chapter Eight for some additional tips on modifying your exercise habits).

No matter what roadblocks you may be dealing with, the important thing is to figure out *why* you're still struggling with them: What old, negative ways of thinking might be influencing your behavior? How can you challenge those thoughts? You know what you need to do to push past your roadblocks, and you have the power to do it.

Write a letter to yourself from an important time in your life (when you felt bad about your body or yourself, when you started to diet, when you were at a low point with your eating disorder, etc.). Tell yourself how your life is going to improve as long as you continue to upcycle and recover (or how it already has!). Tell yourself about all of the things you have to be proud of, such as things you like about your personality, things you are good at, achievements, etc. Tell yourself how you are going to get through that difficult moment, and on with your life. Be creative, and go with whatever it is you are feeling as you write. You know better than anyone else just exactly what you need to say—and hear!

Don't get disheartened if you still find yourself dealing with some of your disordered thoughts and behaviors even well into your recovery. Even though they do go away, it can often be a slow and gradual process. You may well experience lapses; the important thing is to just keep your head up, and keep moving forward. *You will make it.*

Cheryl Kerrigan, 41, of Massachusetts, remembers several feelings of liberation throughout her recovery that told her she was headed in the right direction:

> *"I remember the feeling of freedom I would occasionally get during my recovery that told me I was going in the right direction. The feeling would begin in my heart and make its way into my brain, and a sense of freedom and enlightenment would evolve. It made my heart happy and made me smile. That feeling was confirmation that the hard work and pain I was going through in recovery was paying off and was working. It was proof I was moving in the right direction. This feeling would come out of the blue, so it was exciting when I felt it. It was like a pat on the back and a hug all at once; an acknowledgment that I'm going down the right road. I was able to take those moments and file them inside my head and heart and pull them out when I had a hard day and thought I would never recover. I remembered those feelings often to help me through some tough times. As my recovery got stronger those feelings of freedom became more frequent and before I knew it, the feeling stayed around me all the time. It was (is) pure bliss."*

The obsessive thoughts go away when you allow yourself to finally just live your life by being who you really are and getting rid of all the guilt you associate with eating. You start thinking about things you want to do and accomplish during the day instead of what you're going to eat and how much you're going to exercise. I'm a lot less crabby when I'm not giving death looks to my thighs or hungrily watching everyone else eat cake and ice cream that I "can't have" (we won't talk about how friendly I am when I haven't gotten enough sleep!). When my body and I are friends, I have more time to think about writing and I can actually be present in conversations with people.

Alethia, 26, from Arizona said her husband noticed an amazing change in her once she began to recover:

> *"After my husband came home from overseas there was one day in particular that he looked at me and told me I was beautiful—really beautiful; and not only did I believe that he felt that—but I felt amazing when he said it—and I could say thank you, instead of the typical, 'No I look like crap.' He didn't mean it just physically, either: He could see the dynamic shift in my mind and thoughts and attitude—and me being me—and that was what was sooo beautiful."*

Deb K., 43, from North Carolina was surprised by how much her life opened up through recovery:

> *"I had absolutely the nicest of surprises in my life as I recovered, in that all of a sudden I discovered real hopes and dreams inside me, because in recovery, all of the hopes and dreams that I had ever dared imagine had already come to pass! I had achieved them! Before recovery, when people would ask me what my hopes and dreams were, or my goals in life as people sometimes do, I would make up something philanthropic like I'm going to join the peace corps and then go to medical school and take trips to under-developed countries and volunteer there, maybe find a husband that shares these dreams, raise a family, be active in the community, etc...when inside my head, all I could truthfully think of was 1) I dream of the day I am binge/purge free, 2) I want to eat like a 'normal' person where food is just food, and 3) I desire with all of my heart for exercise to be for health and not as a punishment. That was it, the sum total of everything I ever wanted for myself for as long as I could remember until I was 40 years old and had my second extended stay in a residential treatment center—and my life changed forever."*

Lori, 30, from Florida recalled that her whole world seemed to change:

> *"I remember one day, all of a sudden, my world became colorful. It sounds strange, but I remember thinking, 'Wow! That tree is really green.' I looked around and noticed all of the little things I had missed for years. My senses were heightened. I noticed the smell of the fresh cut grass and felt the coolness of the ground. I heard kids laughing. I felt ALIVE."*

Don't let anything you've heard about true recovery being "impossible" become a justification for you to keep holding onto old behaviors; if you believe you can fully recover, you *will.*

Next are your journal questions, followed by this chapter's family segment and the expert Q & A section, with insight from Carolyn Costin, Keesha Broome, and Barbara Truitt.

Journal Questions

1. If I had never had an eating disorder, how would I respond to some of the things that trigger me now? How can I start responding to some of my triggers in healthier ways?

2. If I've experienced a lapse in my recovery: What happened? How was I feeling prior to the lapse? How could I have reacted differently to the situation? How can I prevent this from happening again?

3. What are some of the roadblocks I struggle with? Why might I still be having some trouble in these areas? What concrete things can I do to overcome my roadblocks (For example, eating a portion of lean beef instead of only chicken, or taking a walk in the park instead of always exercising for an exact length of time on the elliptical machine at the gym)?

4. What are some positive experiences I've had throughout my recovery so far? What am I most looking forward to happening as a result of my recovery?

Tips for Friends & Family

Don't be the "police"…

Although it is important that you make sure your loved one is healthy and stable, you probably won't help their situation if they feel like you're watching their every move. Andrea Roe, 28, from British Columbia, Canada said it is important to not try to change your loved one:

> *"Don't force them to act 'normal.' Just support them. You cannot force them to change their beliefs or behaviors. You cannot force an anorexic to eat, a bulimic to stop vomiting, or a binge eater to stop eating huge amounts of food. Eating disorders are not simply about food and weight."*

But don't be an enabler, either.

Even if you're not monitoring them, also make it clear you won't approve of or accept any of their disordered behaviors. Jenni, 24, from Texas said that the best approach to being supportive is one of balance:

> *"You have to toe the line between being supportive and giving your loved one space. If your loved one feels like you're being too overbearing, she might back away even more. If she feels like you're ignoring her—giving her too much space—she might think she can get away with anything. Let her know you're there for her, and to come to you when she's ready to talk."*

Traci, 37, from California added that it is important to be both caring and firm, so as to not "allow them to manipulate you." Kristen, 25, from Wisconsin said, "Do what you can to accommodate the sufferer, but make sure that someone is keeping them accountable."

Keep a healthy environment.

If your loved one will be living with or staying with you, make sure you have healthy food options and that excess food is put away rather than being left out in the open. If possible, get rid of your bathroom scales or at least put them somewhere they can't easily be accessed.

Watch your words.

Talk with your loved ones about what's helpful for them to hear, and what's not. Ashley Devitt, 18, from Florida said different phrases can often mean different things to different people:

> *"What one may find a compliment, another may take as an insult. For example, I personally like when my parents acknowledge a challenge that I've overcome. I appreciate it when they say, 'I'm proud of you for finishing that meal, Ashley.' However, I know many people who would find that comment extremely offensive."*

How you say something is just as important as what you say: Thecla, 24, from Illinois mentioned friends of hers with the tendencies to say insensitive things at times:

> *"...as much as I am really trying to not pay attention to what I am eating, (they) have to make a comment whenever I eat anything around them. For example, someone will bring cookies into work, and after a battle in my head, I decide that it will be okay for me to have a cookie. Even though I know it will be hard, I decide to go for it. Everyone else is eating cookies; it's really not a big deal. The second I grab the cookie and take a bite, someone will say, 'Oh my gosh, Thecla, you're eating a cookie!' or sometimes I'll even get remarks like, 'Wow, won't that totally go against your diet?' Then, I beat myself up and think I never should have had the cookie to begin with, even if they meant the comment as positive. I wish sometimes they would just ignore that I am eating a cookie, instead of calling all kinds of attention to it."*

Amy Pettengill, 27, from New Hampshire said it's specifically important to not make comments about your loved one's weight:

> *"When someone says, 'You look too thin, sick, gross, unhealthy, etc.,' people with eating disorders might actually take that as a compliment. Also, in early recovery and during the weight restoration process, comments such as, 'You don't look like you have an eating disorder,' or 'You look healthy,' can be taken totally out of context, and perceived as someone saying, 'You look fat.'"*

Please note that I'll talk more about how someone in recovery can respond to triggering comments in Chapter Five.

Reassure me.

Hard work pays off. Help your loved one remember that as long as they just keep at it, they'll see a wonderful new life start to unfold for them!

Questions Friends & Family Should Ask

1. Are there certain foods, comments, or situations that trigger you (cause you to start having unhealthy thoughts)? What can we do to help you when you start to feel triggered?

2. What are some signs that you may be struggling? (For example, talking a lot about weight, cutting food up into tiny pieces, etc.—Review the "How do I know if some of my habits are disordered?" checklist in Chapter One for more potential signs)

3. How can we help create a healthier environment for you?

4. What words and phrases are helpful for you to hear from me? What words and phrases aren't helpful?

Journal Questions for Friends & Family

1. What will I do to help create a healthier environment?

2. How can I help my loved one respond to his/her triggers? What will I do if my loved one doesn't respond in a healthy way?

3. What are some positive things I can say to my loved one? What are some things I should try not to say?

Q & A with Carolyn Costin, MFT, M.A., M.ED., and Keesha Broome, M.A., MFT

Q: How do I keep triggers at bay?

A: Living in today's society, it is highly likely that you will come across people, things, or situations that cause you to doubt yourself or your body. These are triggers—they are everywhere and they are inevitable. A trigger might be directly related to food like dinner at an all-you-can-eat buffet, or it might seem less obvious like a conversation with Mom. But the thing about triggers is, inherently they are not bad. It's ignoring or not understanding them that can lead to trouble. It is useful to identify specific, individual triggers so that when faced with them, you do not fall prey. Once you are aware of and understand your own potential pitfalls, you can better avoid or plan for them in the future. And if a trigger does lead to eating disorder behaviors or a far bigger slip, don't lose hope.

After 15 years of treating clients, I conducted an informal survey among all past clients. I wanted to assess who was doing better and why. Aside from the usual questions regarding their symptoms, I asked them a series of questions about such things as triggers and coping mechanisms. For those who were recovered, there was an amazing similarity among three things most said that they did. I had not realized how significant these tools were. But now, I like to think of myself as sort of "teaching to the test." I tell all of my clients to do these three things to ensure recovery:

1. Journal

Never underestimate the importance of journaling. It's your forum to express your thoughts, uncensored and without fear of judgment. It is also an important way to gain access into your inner conflict. Through journaling, you can tap into your eating disorder self and then talk back to it from your healthy self. You can start by writing down your eating disorder thoughts and bringing your journal into session. Then you, possibly with help from your therapist, can begin writing back to these thoughts. I also encourage my clients to journal at all points of their struggle: when the urges start, in the middle of the behavior, and after they've engaged in their eating disorder. I know it may sound strange, but I tell clients to journal WHILE they are bingeing. Writing down your eating disorder thoughts while they are happening can provide great insight into why and how the ED (eating disorder) voice takes over.

2. Don't Weigh Yourself*

There is never a good enough reason to step on that scale or to know that number. And believe me, I've heard a lot of them. Women in today's culture often unknowingly use the scale as a female torture device. Even when you think you can tolerate what feedback it gives you, and even when you think you'll like the answer, it is a trap. You do not need a number to justify your meal plan or your life. Saying no to the scale is a powerful political act. By releasing the need to know your weight, you are not only liberating yourself and your body but also working to end society's objectification of women. There is no perfect size and no scale that measures spirit. Don't get me wrong, you will need someone keeping track for awhile to let you know you're okay and what's going on in a general sense. But YOU need to stop weighing yourself. Rather than entrusting your safety and well-being to the scale, trust your treatment team. Allow your therapist, dietitian, and/or physician to keep you on track. And begin to believe that you are more than a number.

3. Reach Out for Support

Whether it's a friend, family member, or part of your treatment team, it is critical to reach out to someone as soon as you're feeling bad or like you might want to engage in eating disorder behavior. Asking for help or being honest about your struggles can be hard. People often feel embarrassed or ashamed or think that it's really "not that bad." One way to make it easier is to reach out when things are also going well. Staying connected when life is good can make it much less overwhelming to reach out when it goes bad. I also tell my clients to make a "Red Flags" list that they can share with loved ones. This list consists of behaviors that will signal struggles or a potential relapse. By allowing your support system access to this information, they can better hold you accountable and offer more appropriate support. It is imperative to reach out to your therapist and/or dietitian as soon as you start slipping. This makes it easier to get back on track and helps you steer clear of a more serious situation.

**Note from Justine: You can find more on weighing yourself and finding your healthy weight in Chapter Eight.*

Q: How can I tell if I'm really getting better—or still in denial about some of my behaviors?

A: At my treatment centers, we utilize a level system that, in our estimation, mirrors levels of recovery in the world. On each level, there are certain requirements and also certain privileges that determine where a person is in terms of eating disorder behaviors and thinking. It is an individual's motivation that propels her through this level system. Oftentimes clients are not at a point or do not feel capable of progressing beyond a certain level—a level which might require such things as reaching another weight goal or letting go of certain food behaviors. You might find yourself facing such challenges or feeling stuck at one level of recovery unsure of how to get to the next. This is hitting a Roadblock, and this is okay. It is just where you or someone else may be in recovery.

It is every professional's, and I can venture to say, every family member or loved ones' desire for their person to make a full recovery. Therefore, we will always aim for that goal.

I believe it is possible to be FULLY RECOVERED rather than always being IN RECOVERY. And myself, several of my staff and colleagues around the country, and countless clients around the world, are proof of this possibility. As I discuss in my book *100 Questions and Answers about Eating Disorders*, there are varying definitions of the term recovered. **My definition is when the person can accept his or her natural body size and shape and no longer has a self-destructive or unnatural relationship with food or exercise.** Food has a proper place in life. When you are recovered, you choose what you want, when you want, without fear, restraint, or compensation. You do not use eating disorder behaviors to deal with, distract from, or cope with other problems. When recovered, you will not compromise your health or betray your soul to look a certain way, wear a certain size, or reach a certain number on the scale.

In other illnesses, such as alcoholism or drug addiction, the commonly held belief is that recovery is a continual process—one that requires a person to give up the thing they are having trouble with or abusing. But a person struggling with an eating disorder cannot abstain from that which they abuse—food. Healing from an eating disorder means that food has to be consumed daily, and the individual has to make peace with it, not remove food from his or her life.

And I want to hold this hope for everyone struggling regardless of where they are in their battle. If you have hit a roadblock or have plateaued at a certain level, it is okay. It is important for you to be honest, first and foremost with yourself, about where you are still struggling. **Remember that Red Flags list we mentioned earlier? You should be continually checking it and catching yourself even before others do.** One good honesty check is asking yourself what advice you would give to a peer exhibiting or expressing similar behaviors or thoughts as yours. Would you be alarmed by what they're doing or thinking? Should you be alarmed by the same thoughts or behaviors in which you're engaged?

I will always hold the hope and speak the truth about what life free from an eating disorder looks, feels, and tastes like. And most of the time, a person's own desire to see, feel, and taste it for his or herself helps to spur them forward. Be gentle with yourself as you continue through this process. Roadblocks are not dead ends. Use them to reexamine your path and reevaluate your motivation. Then keep moving down the road of recovery.

Some tips I recommend for getting unstuck:

- Work with a dietitian.
- Focus on what your body can do—NOT what it looks like.
- Remember: Don't weigh yourself—EVER.
- Keep your appointments with your treatment team.
- Incorporate yoga and meditation into your schedule to facilitate rest and mindfulness.
- Be honest about what your thoughts and behaviors really are.

Q & A with Barbara Truitt, RD, LD/N

Barbara Truitt is a registered and licensed dietitian in the state of Florida and has over 23 years of experience in all aspects of clinical nutrition, including in eating disorder inpatient and outpatient programs.

Q: What if I mess up and binge and/or purge?*

A: The rule to keep in mind is to never miss a meal, and never miss a snack. If bingeing and/or purging occur during the day, and your schedule gets interrupted, you pick up where you left off. For example:

7:00 a.m.:	Wake up
8:00 a.m.:	Breakfast
9:00 a.m.:	(Oops, purged) Just because I purged does not mean I get to skip my 10:30 snack—don't restrict!**
10:30 a.m.:	Snack
12:00 p.m.:	Lunch (Oops binged & purged) Move on to your next snack; don't restrict.
3:00 p.m.:	Snack
6:00 p.m.:	Dinner (Oops, purged) Move on to p.m. snack; don't restrict.
9:00 p.m.:	Snack

Also, stick to your meal plan even if you binge without purging! You must do so to try to get back on track. If you don't pick up where you left off in your meal plan, it will be harder to resume your routine. I know it's hard to believe, but just the idea alone can make you think twice about the binge, where before you maybe wouldn't have given it a second thought.

**Notes from Justine: To binge means to eat a larger amount of food in a small period of time than would be expected of others in similar circumstances. Purging can be defined as* *not only vomiting after eating, but also using exercise, laxatives, or diuretics as an attempt to "purge" calories from your body.*

***To restrict means to limit your calories during the day by eating less than your body needs, or to not allow yourself to eat certain foods or food groups.*

3 Please Your Palette:
Rediscovering your self

"I was always looking outside myself for strength and confidence but it comes from within, it is there all the time."

– Anna Freud

As a kindergartener, I was definitely not the kid everyone wanted to play with. I wasn't the boys' favorite girl to chase around the playground at recess (*or* the second or third favorite, for that matter). I was just kind of…there. Sometimes I felt invisible. Other times, I probably would have preferred invisibility: When I was in fourth grade, some of the other girls used to prank call me, to the point where I began to get anxious just from hearing the phone ring.

I never understood what I'd done that made those girls want to do that to me. I don't remember ever tripping any of them at lunchtime or spreading any vicious rumors about them having nasty, highly-contagious skin diseases (even though I sometimes think they might have deserved it a little bit). I spent my time doing things like feeding abandoned kittens milk through eyedroppers, or helping other people with their homework.

By sixth grade, I had subscriptions to all of the most popular teen magazines. As soon as they came in the mail I would run to my room, shut the door, and read every single page from front to back. I'd write down all my favorite tips in the notebook I kept at my side. I was intent that by the time I made it to high school—that flashy, dreamy world I loved to read about—I would know absolutely everything I needed to know in order to be popular. I would be able to start great conversations and make devoted friends. I'd know how to apply my makeup like a supermodel and attract lots of boys. I would be a cheerleader. I would definitely have really nice, shiny hair. By eighth grade, I noticed that some high school guys actually seemed interested in me—after all, I did look a few years older than I really was. I thought for sure that high school was going to be awesome!

I was wrong. High school didn't end up being much better than any of the years before—and in some ways, it was worse. I still didn't have many friends, and the guys my age still treated me a little bit like wallpaper. It wasn't until years after I graduated from *college*, when I ran across a Facebook photo of a bunch of my old classmates, that I had a bit of a revelation. My former classmates were all about four years old in the photo, and all in matching light blue gymnastics uniforms. They were all together. And none of them had ever even met me yet at all.

When I went to kindergarten, I hadn't realized that several of my classmates had known each other well before our first day of school. They had probably been playing together in their backyards for years, while I was living miles out of town and running around in fields with my brother and cousins. Their lack of connection with me throughout those early years wasn't a sign that I was boring or unattractive or some kind of weirdo (okay, well maybe a little bit of that sometimes); they just didn't know me. And because I never developed enough confidence to just be myself, they were never able to get to know the real me.

By the time I was in college, I was an expert at being someone else. I spent my time trying to become the kind of person I thought other people would like, instead of doing any of the things I really loved to do. I was dating someone I had absolutely nothing in common with, other than the school we were going to. My eating disorder was in full swing.

Before I wanted to be thin, I wanted to write. As soon as I learned to read, I started stapling together pieces of scratch paper together and making picture books. When I was in eighth grade, I sat down at our computer and decided I was going to write a novel. I wrote another one my sophomore year, and self-published it before I graduated from high school. Some people at my school started calling me "the next Stephen King," and asking me to autograph copies of my book for them. They thought I was going to go places.

It took me over ten more years to complete another book (this one). Why? Despite my classmates' enthusiasm, I myself began to grow increasingly unsure of my own ability to find real success as a writer. I became anxious every time I sat down at the computer. My fingers would hover over the keyboard, unmoving; words failed me, as self-doubt raced through my mind: *You're wasting your time. You're not writing anything good. Nobody is going to want to read that, or even pay any attention to you.*

When those thoughts began to take over, I would go binge and purge. I didn't have to think about what a failure I thought I was; I could just shut my mind off, and focus on my body. I thought I could control my physical appearance, even if I'd never be able to control the direction in which my life was heading. For awhile, it seemed like the perfect solution.

As my physical appearance became the focus of my identity, I became an empty shell. When you start obsessing over food and your body, you forget about the things you really love to do. Your goals change from getting good grades or getting stronger for your sport, to thinning your thighs. Instead of going out with friends, you might be sitting at home counting calories or trying to figure out how many miles you need to run to "make up" for those extra few bites you took at lunch.

It wasn't until a few years ago, when I began really writing again (to start this book project), that I began to come back to life. I had to upcycle my thoughts, by challenging all my old fears of failure and just start writing again. I began to write for no other reason than because I truly loved to do it—not because I was trying to somehow prove my worth to others by achieving some certain perceived mark of success.

Once I took that pressure off of myself, I started getting excited about waking up in the morning again. It felt good knowing I was *doing* something good. I started to connect with some really wonderful people who encouraged me to keep going. I started to believe that maybe some of the things my ex had been telling me—about how I was weak, and how I needed him just to survive—could be wrong.

One of the most vital aspects of recovery is figuring out what you really care about, and then filling your life with it. Once you do that, you might just find that you don't have room—or need—for your eating disorder anymore. It may just start to fade away!

A life worth living is all about doing what you love, and knowing that you really can do something worthwhile and amazing—you're not just an empty shell. So, how do you bring alive everything that's inside of you?

Say Hello to Yourself

Who are you? Can you answer that?

Right now, make a list of the things that make you who you are: What are some of your favorite things? What do you like to do? What are you good at?

It's essential to **separate yourself from your disorder.** Those habits aren't you; they're a label that stops you from doing what you really want to do. If you're having trouble coming up with answers to the questions above, rewind your life a few (or several!) years and think about yourself when you were a kid: What did you look forward to doing on the weekends when you didn't have school? What made you laugh? What were you good at doing?

Jenni, 24, from Texas started her own separation process simply by making a list of everything she liked about herself:

> *"It sounds silly, and you may not believe the things you're writing at first, but over time you realize that you are valuable—that you're not just a body for ornamentation. With the eating disorder and recovery, I've come full circle with my self-image. Before I got sick, I was happy and confident—I felt great about who I was. Then the eating disorder completely tore me down: I wasn't smart. I wasn't*

pretty. I wasn't a good singer. No one actually liked me (at least, that's what the eating disorder told me). That was a huge struggle for years. During my last treatment, they worked with me a lot on this: They had me make lists of qualities I liked in myself, and they worked with me to discover that I am a whole person. I'm slowly coming to believe those things about myself again: I'm intelligent, I'm kind, I'm artistic, and people aren't just pretending to like me."

Once you've made your list, **create an "All about Me" book.** You can call this a scrapbook if you're a girl (doesn't that sound fun?) or just a book if you're a guy. To get started, make a list of everything you think defines who you are, what you like, and what's important to you: What makes you happy? What annoys you? What makes you laugh? What makes you think? What's your favorite color, movie, book, season, television character, scent, childhood toy, subject in school, etc.? Who was your childhood hero? What's your dream job? What are some of your favorite quotes?

Create as many pages as you'd like with pictures, words, and drawings that relate to all those things on your list. Fill a page with everything that makes you happy. If your favorite color is purple, make a page full of pictures of any fun purple things you can find (grapes, flowers, soccer balls, clothing, whatever!). Make a page devoted to your favorite book, by cutting out pictures of people who you imagine the characters in the book look like, and pictures of things mentioned in the book. If you love winter, make a page with snowmen and mittens and hot cocoa and fireplaces. Make a page with hearts and lots of red and pink if Valentine's Day is your favorite holiday—I think you get the idea!

If you're not exactly the crafty type, don't let that deter you from doing this activity. Your book doesn't have to be fancy or take a lot of time; it can simply be a collection of clippings, photos, notes, and phrases that are meaningful to you. Put everything together in a binder, and feel free to add pages whenever you discover a new passion, hobby, or facet of your personality!

Start filling your time with the things you used to love to do, instead of giving that time to your old unhealthy behaviors. In the middle of my eating disorder, I couldn't think about hobbies. Part of it was because I felt guilty about spending time doing things that were "fun." Part of it was also because some of the eating and exercise habits I had developed had gotten me into such a rut that I didn't have time for anything else. I liked my rut, because it felt comfortable and predictable—like I had some sort of control over my life. However, ruts are paralyzing. It was only when I began to change up my routine and include other fun activities in my life that I began to feel like a real, vibrant person again—*me*. For years, my routine consisted of waking up, thinking about what I was going to eat, meticulously preparing food, eating methodically, working out, thinking about everything I had eaten, calculating and recalculating calories, and thinking about what I would eat and do for exercise the next day. That was it. Maybe it shouldn't be such a surprise to me how much my world has opened up: Now, instead of thinking about those same things all day long, I'm probably thinking about going for a walk with my husband on the path near our house, playing a board game, or writing a new post for my blog, http://youupcycled.com. I feel like there are vibrant colors in my world that I never saw before.

Schedule time for fun just like you schedule work, and don't feel guilty about doing things that make you happy. You deserve to have a fun, happy life, just as much as anyone else. You're a very special person to all kinds of different people. There are things you do that no one else can do. When you're happy and relaxed you're more likely to be productive, think creatively, and feel more confident in your abilities. Your mood affects other people, too: I'm really crabby when I'm not taking some time to do things I like to do. My husband *really* appreciates it when I take some time for myself!

Don't always just stick to what's familiar; **try some new hobbies, too.** Have you ever played tennis or golf? How about scrapbooking or painting? Don't be afraid to start small, with mini-golf or finger-paints. The key is just to *try* something. It will only be a matter of time before you find something you love.

Discover a purpose for yourself. Your whole life changes once you recognize something you want to do and start figuring out how you can use your talents and abilities to do it. Besides writing and speaking, I decided to go back to school to earn my graduate degree in counseling to help other people with disordered eating, unhealthy relationships, and some of the other challenges I've encountered in my own life. It feels good to know that I might be able to make a difference somehow, and as a potential role model for others, I'm motivated to always take care of myself.

How do you discover your purpose? You might begin to find it as you start doing the things you love to do again, or as you begin to try new things. If you're interested in exploring some volunteer opportunities in your area, http://www.volunteermatch.org is a great place to start.

Your purpose will become clearer once you learn to **listen to your Self.** This is one of the most powerful things you can do in your life. Truth speaks inside of you, but you have to learn to differentiate it from all of the *other* voices that get in its way: Every day of your life, you're getting countless messages from the media, your family, friends, and even random people you overhear at the grocery store or wherever else. People all have their own ideas about things, whether that be related to dieting and body image or even careers, relationships, or morality—no matter what the topic, everyone has their own opinions and they're usually more than happy to give them to you. You've probably internalized other people's ideas, simply because you've heard them so often. I listened to some of the girls I went to high school with talk about dieting so much that I began to think being thin was important for me, despite having loved my own natural curves very much earlier on. After reading too many articles about low-carb diets, I developed an irrational fear of carbohydrates.

As I said in Chapter One, I call all of the swirling negative influences around us the "Peanut Gallery": There will always be plenty of messages around to distract and mislead you, but none of the people spreading those messages have a clue what's right for *you.* At the end of the day, it's up to you to look inside yourself and discover the truth—even if you have to do some digging. What is *your* voice saying? Keep in mind that I'm not talking about the *negative* voice that's inside of you; *that* negative voice is actually the most debilitating member of the Peanut Gallery. That negative voice develops out of your own fears and insecurities, and it grows stronger as you listen to other people who say things that make your fears and insecurities worse.

Look inside for validation. Don't live your life trying to gain approval from other people. Even though constructive feedback can be really helpful when you're trying to do something like fine-tune your resume or develop a presentation for work, there's no one in the world who can tell you how to *be you*; you're the only one who knows how to do that. It may take some time and exploration, but you'll figure it out. Just be completely honest with yourself, give a real effort in everything you do, and *trust yourself.*

Create a daily reminder. Arielle Lee Bair, 27, from Pennsylvania said she programmed her cell phone alarm to go off (silently) each morning at 9 a.m., with a special reminder message:

> *"'I like myself.' That's what my phone tells me to remember. Sometimes we all need reminding...if you don't like yourself yet, just wait. A few weeks of seeing that daily message and it might start to sink in."*

Make a list of your goals and keep it somewhere you'll always be able to see it. Include both recovery goals (like eating a fear food or reaching your first anniversary of being in recovery) and life goals (like earning a college degree or being a positive role model to your neice or nephew) on your list, and look at it whenever you feel like you're getting off track. Andrea Roe, 28, from British Columbia, Canada kept a list of her goals glued to the mirror in her room to keep herself focused on them instead of her eating disorder. She said it was rewarding to look back at it later and see how many of her goals she actually accomplished.

If you're a hands-on type of person, go one step further and **make a "Hopes Board."** Get a large magnetic or pin board and put it up in your room. Whenever you come across quotes, tips, photos, or any objects that inspire you or represent things you want to accomplish, stick them up on the board so you'll be able to see them when you wake up and before you go to sleep. Rearrange and add to the board regularly so it stays fresh and doesn't start to just blend into the wallpaper for you. Use the board to start thinking about some of the goals you want to create and begin accomplishing in the activity below:

Make a plan to achieve your goals. Once you begin focusing on all of the wonderful things you want to do with your life, you'll notice your disordered behaviors gradually beginning to take a backseat. Just don't let yourself get overwhelmed thinking about how you're going to accomplish them! Sit down with someone whose opinion you respect (like a counselor, pastor, therapist, coach, or mentor) and figure out which goals you want to work on first: Is there a specific career field you want to get into someday? Do you want to start a volunteer group in your community? Have you been dreaming of writing a novel? Spend some time brainstorming ways you could go about reaching your goals, one at a time. Choose three of your best options for achieving each goal, and then ask yourself the following regarding each of those options:

1. How difficult would this path be for me?

2. How likely is it that this path will help me accomplish my goal?

3. What are all of the possible positive outcomes of taking this path?

4. What are some potential drawbacks to this path?

Analyze your answers for each option, and then based on those answers, choose which route you would like to pursue. Then, start figuring out what specific steps you can begin completing on the path towards your goal. You can do this by asking yourself the following questions:

1. How long might it take (realistically) to accomplish this goal?

2. What smaller goals will I need to accomplish in order to reach the larger goal?

3. What would I like to have accomplished within one month? Six months? One year?

4. What can I try to accomplish this week related to my goal?

5. What can I do today to begin working toward my goal?

6. What challenges might I face in trying to reach my goal? What will I do when I face one of these challenges?

Once you've spent some time thinking and journaling about your answers to those questions, start making a plan of action. Use those people you trust as sounding boards for your ideas, and do your research by learning everything you can about what you want to do, including talking to people who have done similar things. Commit to spending a little time *every day* working on one of your small goals. Buy a nice planner and actually write down things you want to do each day, along with the times when you'll do them. When that scheduled time comes, protect yourself from any distractions that may get in the way, like phone calls, the comfy couch that's just begging you to take a nap, or (especially) self-doubt. The key to success is remembering that there is never one set path to achieving the things you really want to do—results come from dedication and persistence.

Start a special interest group. Do you have a passion that you want to share with others? Would you like to meet other people with a common interest? Whether you have an affinity for cooking international foods, gardening, playing street hockey, or salsa dancing, there are probably other people out there who would love to join you! Getting a group started can be as simple or as complex as you want it to be. Here are some basic steps to get your group off the ground:

1. Determine what, specifically, you want your group to be for: Is it a general cooking group, or only for specific kinds of foods? Will people actually be cooking at the group meetings, or will they be bringing recipes and foods for others to taste?

2. Find a location for your group. If you're planning on keeping things simple and just having a few friends meet up regularly to knit blankets for needy children, meetings can be held in someone's home. However, if you're planning on having yoga classes and inviting people you don't know, it may be more conducive to have gatherings somewhere like the multipurpose room of an office building or in a school gymnasium (after you obtain permission from the administrators of these places of course!).

3. Decide how often, when, and how long you will meet specifically: Are you going to get together on Tuesday evenings from 7 to 8 p.m., every other Saturday morning from 10 a.m. until 1 p.m., or every 3rd Monday over the lunch hour?

4. Think about who you would like to have involved in your group: Friends? Friends of your friends? People from your church, school, or place of employment? Anyone in the community?

5. Figure out how you will let people know about the group: Will you simply invite some of your friends, and tell your friends to tell their friends about it? Will you post notices in your church bulletin, local newspaper, workplace newsletter, or through your social media accounts? What other free or inexpensive methods of getting the word out can you utilize?

Don't get disheartened if your group doesn't seem to be thriving right away; often, it just takes time for things to build. As long as you stay committed it will only be a matter of time before you start to see your group begin to grow!

Don't back down from your dreams. As nerve-wracking as it may be, **the best thing you can do when you're feeling anxious or doubtful is just keep moving toward your goals, step by step**. As long as you keep facing forward, in time you *will* begin to see results. Once that happens you'll notice a whole new attitude, and your old unhealthy habits will begin to lose their hold on you. It hasn't been easy for me to write this book; as I said, I had to work through a whole bunch of writing-related anxiety to get where I am today. I've learned that when I write, I can't overanalyze every single thing on the page to the point where I can't even put two words together. I have to stay focused on my real intent, instead of imagining what all of the critics out there will say. I won't be able to accomplish what I'm working for if I keep beating myself up or distracting myself before I can actually do it. The editing can come later.

Dr. Diana Repack, 46, from Pennsylvania was amazed by what she was able to do once she let go of her eating disorder label and started embracing her goals:

> *"I thought I was my eating disorder and my eating disorder was me. When I started to think about really giving it up, I wondered what would be left of me. I feared that nothing would be interesting about me. In reality, what I found was that the more I gave up the eating disorder, the more interesting I actually became. People didn't have to listen to me whine about feeling 'fat' or what I had to eat that day; instead, I could have conversations about other things—things that I only found time and energy for when I started letting go of the eating disorder. And as a compulsive over-exerciser, I also freed up a lot of time when I learned that I could get a heck of a lot more accomplished at the gym in one hour than I was accomplishing in three times that. I did so many things I never would have done if I had not given up the eating disordered behaviors. I got my private pilot license, I earned an M.B.A. and a Doctorate degree, and right now, I am a few weeks away from testing*

for my Black Belt in Tang Soo Do Karate. Believe me, you will find other things to do once you free yourself from the prison of an eating disorder—things you will enjoy."

Like Diana, **you'll be better equipped to achieve your goals the further along you get in your recovery.** Hilary Crist, 27, from California recognized a total transformation in her ability to think once she separated from her disorder:

"Recovery has freed my thoughts from the prison that they were trapped in. Having your mind free from obsessive eating disorder thoughts can only be described as exhilarating. I was completely consumed with thoughts about food and my body. Once my mind was free, I was able to begin on the road of self-discovery about me—Hilary—what I liked to do, the dreams and aspirations I had for the future, places I wanted to travel, etc. My return of my concentration and focus was, and still is, priceless."

Alexandra, 23, from Sussex, England, began a new career during her recovery. She said that as a professional harpist, she didn't have the strength or concentration to play until she got healthier. She said she never would have been able to perform if she was still starving herself. Ellen, 26, from New York discovered a passion for writing that she now can't imagine living without.

Throughout every moment, **have faith.** Trust your own abilities, and if you're a religious person, trust in God's plan for you. Faith will serve you on your best and worst days, and on every day in between. On my good days, I thank God for opening my heart and giving me opportunities to spend my life doing things that are meaningful for me. On my bad days, I pray for strength and the ability to know which steps to take next. Every day, I pray for a more open heart so that I may hear what God is trying to say to me about myself, my life, and where to go next. I also always pray for patience and the ability to appreciate my life as it is *now*, remembering that everything will happen in its right time.

I will never forget a very critical moment in my life, in the middle of the night, when I began to fear that everything I had ever known about life and God could be wrong: It was my first night after leaving that horrible relationship I mentioned in Chapter One, and I was alone in a bed at my parents' house. To say I was confused about what was going on would be one of the world's hugest understatements. I had never missed going to church on Sunday. I tried to pray the Rosary every day. I had had a *plan* for my life, and I prayed for that plan every single night. But at that moment, I feared I might never actually have a single one of the things I wanted most—a husband, a family, or a fulfilling career.

Hadn't God been listening? Was He even really there at all?

Somewhere amidst all my praying, I had missed that critical step of having faith. When I began being honest with myself, I knew that over the past few years I had been living my life according to what *I* thought I "should do" and what I thought needed to happen at certain specific times, instead of listening to God and my heart. I ignored all the thoughts I'd had about my relationship being wrong, simply because I'd thought it was "time" to be in a relationship. I'd had deadlines for myself that I didn't want to miss. But by trying to force certain things to happen at the wrong times and in the wrong ways, I ended up throwing my whole life off course for awhile.

Thankfully, the damage wasn't permanent. I learned my lesson and I'm happy to say that things are now better than ever: A couple of years after the lowest point of my life, after I'd had time to learn and heal and grow, I met my husband Todd (I'll tell you all about that in Chapter Five!). I didn't meet him until I began finally just trusting God and His plan for me. Nowadays, whenever I start to worry, all I have to do is think about my husband. Even though there was once a time in my life when I thought I might never find anyone, I'm now with someone who is as perfect for me as humanly possible. It didn't happen until I learned what faith really is!

Sharon, 32, from Nova Scotia, Canada, said that now that she's recovered, she feels like a whole person with a new lease on life:

> *"I'm a dynamic and complete person. I'm intelligent, creative, fun, happy, and beautiful. I am able to apply knowledge learned in one area to another with greater ease than before. New dimensions have opened up for me, and opportunities seem to never stop falling into my lap. I'm ready for what the world has to offer me. I'm positive about what's coming my way. I know that I can handle it, because I've come so far. I often think I should have been dead by now, but somehow I'm not…and that's a reason to celebrate. If I can keep that mindset, I can do anything. I will continue to do pretty much anything, not bogged down by a weight-obsession or a need to please the world."*

Troy Roness, 23, from North Dakota, said that he has grown tremendously throughout his own recovery:

> *"Everyone around me always says, 'Hey, Troy! It's the old you again!' And in my head I am thinking to myself, 'They have no idea how wrong they are!' I laugh the same, I have my affect back, I talk and just LIVE life again. But, it isn't the 'old' Troy, it's a newer, happier, and more REAL one—a guy who is becoming more comfortable with himself every day, and who isn't ashamed of showing everything that the 'old' Troy never let anyone see. Before, he tried to entertain everyone else's wants and standards, and never his own. This time around, Troy is choosing his own path to take, and he isn't looking back."*

Even if there isn't a single positive thing you can think of to say about yourself right now, strive to view yourself as a survivor rather than someone with an eating disorder. Arielle Lee Bair, 27, from Pennsylvania discovered that simply being in recovery made her feel much more special than having an eating disorder ever did:

> *"I was one of those people who thought that being the skinny (or skinniest) girl was my identity—that having an eating disorder to hold on to made me special. Not so. I was mistaken. I realized, after plodding along on the recovery path for awhile, that I was in fact MUCH more special for embarking on the new journey than for deciding to continue a life of suffering and destruction. I realized that I was brave. Bold. Determined in a way that took more willpower than anorexia did. It was refreshing, but it was also empowering."*

You've probably put a lot of time and effort into your eating disorder; now is your chance to put that time and effort toward discovering, accepting, and developing your *self.* Once I started finally just being myself, I began to notice that people would smile when I walked into a room—something both surprising and amazing to me. I learned that I'm actually good at making people laugh, even if they're having a bad day, and that I really do have some wonderful things to contribute to the world. Like you, I have strengths and abilities that I would never be able to fully explore if I was still trying to become a carbon-copy of other people.

Use your willpower for something *positive.* Concentrate on finally letting yourself *be* yourself and do what it is that you are gifted at doing. Don't get overwhelmed by how daunting some of your goals may seem, or let fear-of-failure stop you. You'll get there.

Next are this chapter's journal questions, followed by the family section and a touching journal excerpt from a contributor.

Journal Questions

1. How would I describe myself to someone I don't know very well yet? For example: What do I like to do for fun? What am I good at doing? What am I passionate about?

2. What dreams do I have for myself? How might my eating disorder be holding me back from accomplishing those dreams?

3. Where do I want to see myself next year (recovery-related or otherwise)? What kinds of things can I do to get myself there?

4. How will I feel about myself, my new lifestyle, and everything I've accomplished, once I'm not struggling with my eating disorder

anymore?

Tips for Friends & Family

Don't focus on the disorder.

Try to focus on your loved one as a person, rather than always thinking about their eating disorder. What are their special qualities? What are they good at? The more time they spend developing their talents and abilities, the less time they will have to focus on food and body issues.

Don't refer to your loved one as being "anorexic" or "bulimic"; those are labels that don't define who he or she is as a person. Instead, say that they are battling or dealing with anorexia or bulimia.

Shannon, 22, from Texas said it bothers her when people who want to become part of her recovery continually ask her questions about it. She said, "I mean my goal is to be normal, and if I am always questioned about my disorder, then I can't just go out with friends and forget about it and just be that normal girl. My closest friends respect that, and wait until I bring the disorder up."

Andrea Roe, 28, from British Columbia, Canada said family and friends should encourage their loved ones to do activities with them, like take a walk, go shopping, spend time on hobbies, or just have a meaningful conversation.

Understand that your loved one may change.

You may notice a bit of a difference in your loved one's personality through recovery, which is usually a good thing. Ashley Devitt, 18, from Florida, pointed out that sometimes disorders mask personal characteristics: "When I was in therapy, my parents kept saying they wanted the 'old me' back, but it's important to recognize that the 'old me' was a sweet, compliant girl who never spoke up. After therapy, I was not the same passive girl as I was before, and I wanted my parents to recognize that."

Questions Friends & Family Should Ask

1. What are your favorite qualities about yourself?

2. What do you see yourself doing in five years? Ten years? What

dreams do you have for yourself once you recover?

3. What kinds of things do you enjoy doing that we can do together?

Journal Questions for Friends & Family

1. What are my favorite things about my loved one? What are some of their positive abilities and qualities that I'd like to share with them?

2. How can I encourage my loved one to keep working towards his or her goals?

3. What are some things I enjoy doing with my loved one? When can we do some of them?

Contributor Journal Excerpt

August 11, 2006

"... I have learned from treatment that, like recovery, many things experienced in life are a process. The joy is in the beginning steps, the journey, and finally the destination. It is all valuable, kind of like the growing of a child: the pregnancy, the birth, each new learned skill, increase in size and awareness, to adolescence and adulthood. The process of a human life, it is all part of the existence. I have either not taken or have missed many of the steps of my journey, my process. And while I cannot replace those missed or untaken steps, or start over, I can learn from what I have missed, from the wrong path that I chose and go forward, new and excited with anticipation of what may lie ahead. And I now know that I have a purpose, a special talent or gift, or place to be where I will be fulfilled."

-- Jody Lanham, 55, Ohio

4 Eat Mindfully: Improving your emotional atmosphere

"The longer I live, the more I realize the impact of attitude on life. Attitude, to me, is more important than facts. It is more important than the past, than education, than money, than circumstances, than failures, than successes, than what other people think or say or do. It is more important than appearance, giftedness, or skill. It will make or break a company…a church…a home.

"The remarkable thing is we have a choice every day regarding the attitude we will embrace for that day. We cannot change our past…we cannot change the fact that people will act in a certain way. We cannot change the inevitable.

"The only thing we can do is play on the one string we have, and that is our attitude…I am convinced that life is 10% what happens to me and 90% how I react to it. And so it is with you."

-- *Charles Swindoll*

Every once in awhile, when I'm sitting in church, I start thinking about passing out. I'll be singing away to "God Bless America" or "One Bread, One Body," or even just listening to the sermon, and then I'll start to feel a little bit woozy. I'll start to imagine myself falling over and clunking my head against the pew, or knocking my husband and everyone else next to him down like a row of dominoes. Everyone in the church will stare at me because that's what people in church do, and then every time I come to church for the rest of my life people will stare at me and wonder if I'm going to pass out. And every time I walk through the church doors, I'll be worrying about passing out so I don't become known as the "Fainting Goat Girl" (you know, like those goats that pass out every time they're startled?).

My worries about fainting aren't due to any health complications; I'm happy to say that I'm actually quite healthy nowadays. But I do still deal with anxiety from time to time—mostly because I'm a daydreaming writer so I don't have the world's longest attention span. I think enough of my anxiety is due to the simple fact that I like to keep my mind occupied, so if I'm waiting in line at the grocery store and reading the headlines of the tabloids isn't doing it for me, I might start to think about passing out (or I might start thinking about which ninja moves I'll use to fight off the person behind me who I imagine is giving me funny looks). I should also mention the fact that I've developed a "special" habit of holding my breath just a little bit when I start to get nervous or stressed out—hence the lightheadedness that often sparks my anxiety in the first place!

One of the biggest keys for me in learning to identify and respond to my emotions has definitely been awareness of my own body. When I start to feel emotional, besides thinking about what specifically is happening *around* me to make me feel that way, I pay close attention to how I'm feeling physically. I've learned that a lot of the things you feel when you start to get anxious are simply your body's reactions to stress. When your body perceives stress, its response is essentially to go into "Fight or Flight" mode: Your heart starts to pound and blood goes to your extremities as your body prepares to act. When this happens, you'll inevitably feel lightheaded. Your fingers and toes might feel tingly, and your stomach might be upset. If you don't understand what's going on, any of these feelings—the pounding heart, dizziness, nausea—can make a little bit of anxiety or stress turn into full-blown panic.

It might sound a little crazy, but now that I'm aware of my body's physical reactions, I actually feel okay when I notice my heart starting to beat a little faster in the grocery store checkout line. Instead of worrying that something is wrong with me, I'm able to remind myself that it's just a bit of anxiety…and that it'd probably be a great idea to start breathing again.

That's not to say you shouldn't pay attention to the mental part of those emotions; there might be significant reasons for them that you need to address. When I had an eating disorder, I used to have panic attacks because I knew I was doing something very bad for me, without anyone else having any idea what was going on. The anxiety didn't go away until I told my family the truth and began getting better. Like me, many of your emotions have causes that you'll need to discover and understand. It is also of key importance to be able to manage your emotions *before* they get out of control. I've learned to recognize and respond to my anxiety before it turns into a full-blown panic attack, because I understand all of the physiological reasons behind some of the scary physical feelings (heart pounding, palms sweating, etc.).

Now, when my church daydreaming goes awry and I start to think about which direction I should fall when I pass out, so as to avoid a serious concussion, I upcycle my thoughts by challenging myself. I'll say something like, "So what if I pass out? That just means I'll get to take it easy the rest of the day, curled up with my fuzzy blanket on the couch and watching Disney movies."

I don't ever pass out—and then I get to spend the day cleaning the bathroom or doing laundry or something (yay?).

I started challenging my fears once I began learning more about Cognitive Behavioral Therapy, or CBT—something I highly recommend to anyone, no matter what their emotions are like on a daily basis. As I mentioned in this book's introduction, CBT basically teaches you that all of your feelings result from your thoughts. Your thoughts can be spurred by either something that happens to you, or something you feel physically. If I have a negative thought, I'll *feel* negative emotionally: For example, if I feel lightheaded because I'm singing a string of high notes without taking a breath, and think to myself, "You're going to pass out,"—I'm going to feel afraid. However, if I have a positive thought, I'm going to have a positive emotion: I might remind myself that I'm lightheaded because I need to breathe more, and then I'll feel fine. With CBT, you start recognizing your thought patterns and learn to upcycle your negative thoughts—which helps you start having a better outlook!

Thanks to CBT, my upcycling philosophy, and a whole lot of self-discovery, these days I consider myself to actually be more emotionally aware than most people: I keep tabs on how I'm feeling throughout the day and I'm usually able to figure out what I need to do to remedy some of my more negative emotions, like getting enough sleep, staying away from caffeine (which is a major cause of anxiety and panic for many people), and breathing every once in awhile! Later in this chapter I'll share some of the things I did to become more emotionally aware.

But first, here are some other tips you can use to start feeling better soon!

The Secrets to Feeling Good

The first secret to feeling good emotionally shouldn't be that big of a surprise: **Make sure you're eating well and treating your body right.** This means balancing your exercise with plenty of rest and eating enough to keep your body happy and your mind sharp. It wasn't until I started eating normally and reached a healthy weight that my emotions felt more normal too. I still get a little cranky when I'm hungry sometimes, but it happens much more gradually than it used to. I also am able to think a lot more easily now, which comes in really handy when you're trying to write a book—or do anything, for that matter! It's amazing how much better you feel when your body and brain have the nutrition they need in order to function properly (Check out Chapter Six for some specifics on meal planning).

Next, **start paying attention to what you're feeling on the inside—** and remember that "fat" isn't a real feeling! The next time you start to criticize your body, think about what was going on right before you started to feel that way: Were you thinking about something stressful or sad? Were you feeling a little overwhelmed or frustrated by something? Telling yourself that you "feel fat" can be a mask for emotions you're not sure how to deal with. Rayna, 26, from Ohio, said it wasn't until she stopped allowing herself to answer "fat" when someone asked her how she was feeling that she learned to figure out what was really going on inside her.

Learning to identify and respond to emotions can pose a special challenge for males. Patrick Bergstrom, 26, from Maryland, said that many men feel that it is unacceptable for them to express their feelings:

> *"Men experience the pressure to become bigger, faster, and stronger by nature. We are supposed to be the caretakers of the home, and not show emotion, fear, or pain. Men don't cry nor do we share our feelings. We put up walls or defenses and avoid conflict and issues dealing with personal feelings."*

Whether you're a man or a woman, it may take a little bit of practice before you start figuring out what's going on inside you. It was helpful for Shana, 24, from Ohio, to **use one of those posters with faces and emotions on it to begin giving names to feelings.** You can also **use a journal to begin exploring your emotions:** When you start to feel something negative, write about what you were doing and what you were thinking shortly before you began to feel that way. This can help you get at the root of what you're experiencing. The simple act of putting your feelings on paper is a great way to get your emotions "out" of you. Some other helpful releases are drawing, painting, listening to music, walking, or anything else that will help you get rid of some of that negative energy (If you haven't already, make sure you see the "Alternative Activity" list idea in Chapter One).

Pinpoint your emotional triggers. When you find yourself feeling icky, pay attention to what was going on beforehand. Like me, you may find that you feel worse after you've had caffeine, because of some of the physical effects it can have on your body, like restlessness, nervousness, or a rapid heartbeat. If you're not breathing properly, you probably will feel lightheaded or fatigued. Lack of sleep will cause you not only to feel physically drained, but also less able to handle emotional distress. In my case, even though I wasn't aware of it for awhile, feeling tired was even more of a trigger for me because the physical sensations associated with it actually reminded me of how I always felt right around the time my bad relationship ended—an incredibly painful period of time for me, when I had a lot of trouble sleeping. If you've gone through something traumatic, there may be certain sounds, feelings, sights, or scents that trigger some pretty uncomfortable feelings for you as well. It's important to recognize what those things are so that you can learn how to respond to them.

When you start to feel a negative emotion, take some time to write about what was going on in your life immediately prior to that emotion: Where were you at? What were you doing? What were you thinking?

Once you've answered those questions, spend some time going over your answers and see if anything sticks out to you as to why you may have started feeling poorly (again, this is an area where a therapist would be very helpful). Just understanding why you felt the way you did will help you begin to manage your emotions and, often, also figure out what you may be able to do to prevent yourself from feeling that way in the future.

A counselor or therapist can give you an objective, educated perspective on some of your thought patterns and what kinds of things you can do to improve them. I know you've probably heard it said about a thousand times that eating disorders aren't about food; with your counselor, you can start figuring out how to work through what really *is* going on. Your counselor can help you cope with specific emotional difficulties, like depression, anxiety, panic attacks, or anger. He or she will also be able to help you figure out some emotion-related goals for yourself, as well as what kinds of things you can do to start accomplishing those goals.

Make sure your counselor is a good fit for you: Different people have different styles, so you might not click with the first (or second, or third!) person you meet with. That doesn't mean counseling isn't right for you; it just means you need to find someone else. It probably will be more helpful if you can work with someone who has experience with eating disorders, but it isn't an absolute requirement, as long as your counselor is willing to educate himself or herself about what you're going through. Again, the biggest thing is just making sure you have a good rapport with one another.

Beyond your counselor, **remember who's in your corner.** Keep a list of phone numbers of other people you can call when you need to talk, like friends and family who are supporting you. Even though you are ultimately the one who is responsible for your own happiness and well-being, it's important to have people in your life you can count on when you just need to talk or hear a friendly voice.

Upcycle your negative thoughts. One of the components of Cognitive Behavioral Therapy (CBT) is keeping a daily thought record, so you can pay more attention to your thought patterns. As I said earlier, CBT teaches that the thoughts you have affect your moods, which thereby affect your behaviors. For example: If you walk into a room thinking, "Everyone is looking at the ketchup stain on my shirt," you're probably not going to feel very good when you enter that room. It's going to affect the way you feel, and the way you act. If you act self-conscious, people probably aren't going to respond as well to you. Their responses will just continue to fuel your negative thoughts.

If, on the other hand, you walk into a room thinking something like, "There's a tiny stain on my shirt, but it's not a big deal because we have more important things to talk about," you're going to feel and act like the type of person *you* want to be. By changing that one little thought, you're going to have a much different experience.

So how can you develop a *better* cycle? The following activity is one I highly suggest you do with a therapist or counselor if possible: Make copies of the template on the following page, or create a larger five-column table in your word processor. If you'd like, you could also draw something similar in your journal.

Start paying attention when you feel stressed, anxious, self-conscious, depressed, angry, etc. during the day, and write down that feeling in the first column.

In the second column, write down what you were thinking immediately before you started feeling that way (this will take practice, but you'll get better at recognizing those thoughts the more you pay attention to them).

Third, write down what happened that spurred that thought: What were you doing at the time? Who else was there? What happened, and what was said?

Fourth, write down a more positive thought that can act as an effective counter to the negative thought. Remember that this can't just be any positive affirmation—it has to be a good, solid statement that you actually believe. If you want, have a friend, family member, or your therapist help you come up with some counter-thoughts.

Last, write how you think that new, more positive thought will make you feel. Once you begin actually getting the chance to try out your "rewritten" thoughts, record how you actually feel after using them.

Keep your binder or notebook with you and make a conscious effort to recognize and rewrite your thoughts on a daily basis.

Your thought record will help you begin to observe patterns in the way you think, enabling you to adapt those patterns and gradually change your whole outlook. Give it some time and real effort, and I promise that you will start to think *and* feel in an entirely new and better way!

CBT has seriously changed my life. When something happens to me now, I'm much more aware of my own thought patterns. When I start to worry that my husband might have gotten into a horrible car accident because he isn't home on time, I'm able to redirect my thoughts by reminding myself that he is probably just finishing up a project or picking up something from the grocery store on his way back.

See the following page for an example of what your thought record should look like:

"Rewriting Negative Thoughts" Journal Page

Negative Feeling	Negative Thought	Preceding Event	Positive Replacing Thought	Resulting Feeling
Example: Anxious. Ashamed.	I'm such an idiot.	I forgot what I was trying to say during my speech.	I stumbled a bit, but I made some good points.	Slightly embarrassed but okay.

If you're interested in learning more about CBT, talk to your counselor or check out some of the resources I have listed in the back of the book.

Stop destructive thoughts. When I was in my counseling internship, I worked with a 4th grade girl who had anxiety. We read through a book called *What to Do When You Worry Too Much: A Kid's Guide to Overcoming Anxiety,* by Dawn Huebner. The technique from the book that worked best for her was pretending the worries she had were little monsters that she could flick off of her shoulders, tell to shut up, and squish with her feet. She actually began to smile when I asked her about her worries, because she was thinking about how she liked to beat them up so they couldn't bother her anymore!

The same sort of concept has worked for me when I've found myself dealing with a lot of unnecessary anxiety: Because I know that all of that excessive worrying does nothing but make me feel worse, I do well with saying something like, "Knock it off. You're fine," and then getting busy with a project or visiting with a friend. If I'm nervously waiting to see the doctor or dentist, I take my phone along with me so I can play solitaire or a word game, rather than letting my mind wander while I page through one of the magazines there. I started doing this after I read the book *The 10 Best-Ever Anxiety Management Techniques*, by Margaret Wehrenberg (a book I highly recommend!), and it's done wonders in terms of reducing my anxiety in certain situations. **If you have a smartphone, download a couple of games that will keep your concentration the next time you're nervously awaiting an appointment, or simply having trouble staving off anxious thoughts.** If you don't have a smartphone, pick up a word search book or some other kind of puzzle book. It's hard to ruminate on your worries when you're focused on figuring out solutions to those games and puzzles.

Upcycle your environment. As I mentioned in Chapter One, when I was going through a stressful period and having trouble sleeping a few years ago, I asked my family to help me move around the furniture in my bedroom. The new look in that space really helped me begin to sleep better! I *felt* different (less stressed) because the environment I was sleeping in *looked* different. In that "new" space, it was also easier for me to practice some of the relaxation methods I was learning, without automatically reverting back to all of those negative thoughts that had been keeping me awake. It was easier for me to get a new start once I felt like I was physically in a new place.

A little redecorating can do a lot of good for your recovery. Ask for a little help rearranging the furniture in your living space. Your new environment will help you feel like the new person you are working to become!

Don't be afraid to feel your feelings. Have you seen that commercial where they say "Depression hurts"? I never understood it until I actually became so depressed that it physically *did* hurt. It felt like my heart was literally aching. I felt weak and tired, and my mind was constantly foggy (magnified even more by my sleep deprivation).

Much of the reason you developed disordered eating and exercise behaviors in the first place may be because you were trying to avoid difficult feelings. However, no matter how awful some of those emotions can be, you have to let yourself feel them in order to be able to work through them. Things might feel a little raw and harsh at first, and you might feel vulnerable without the "security blanket" your eating disorder provided. As tough as it is, it's only once you begin to let yourself actually feel all your feelings that you learn they don't last forever. They're completely normal, and it's even possible to turn them into something positive. For example, feeling unhappy or anxious can be a sign that you need to change something in your life, or even just do something fun to distract yourself or refocus for a bit. The more aware you become of your own emotions, the better you'll be at figuring out exactly what you need to do to make yourself feel better. Again, **a therapist or counselor will be immensely valuable in helping you sort out some of your toughest emotions—don't try to do it all on your own!**

Laura R., 30, from New York, still vividly remembers the day she first truly began experiencing her emotions. It was the same day she realized she could overcome anorexia:

> *"It was Christmas Eve 2006, the anniversary of my mom's death. I was incredibly sad and missing her terribly. Instead of restricting, I made the choice to eat all three meals that day—and snacks, too! It was the first time that I ate despite—and while—experiencing intense emotions. Eating helped me to feel calm, which was a new sensation. Because I wasn't focused on being hungry, I allowed myself to miss my mom, even though it was painful. I cried and felt better afterwards. It was a true breakthrough! I know my mom was watching over me and was proud of me."*

No matter what you're dealing with, you can learn to respond to your emotions in a healthy way. It does take a bit of practice, and it's never exactly easy—but it does get easi*er*.

Ground yourself when dealing with emotions related to bad memories. Lori, 30, from Florida, said she used grounding techniques to help her bring herself back to the present. She suggested finding something in your surroundings that "uses each sense," by asking yourself these questions:

1. What three things do you see?

2. What do you hear?

3. What do you smell?

4. What do you feel (for example, are you sitting on a chair or standing on the ground)?

Once you've answered these questions, reflect on your answers and remind yourself that you are no longer in that difficult moment. Please also be aware that if you struggle recurrently with bad memories, it would be best to visit with a therapist or counselor about them. He or she will be able to help you examine your feelings related to these experiences and hopefully figure out how to begin moving on from them.

Patrick Bergstrom, 26, from Maryland, said he learned to **use laughter in times of difficulty.** He said that although he had always been known to be funny, his eating disorder stole that from him. Throughout treatment, he recovered his sense of humor and used it to help both himself and others:

> *"Therapy can be quite intense, but throwing in a few jokes can really make it pretty painless. My brother's wife never knew me without my eating disorder, but when she saw me after treatment, she was like, 'Wow Patty, you are so funny.' For so long I had lost my swagger, but I got it back and I am smiling all the time. Laughter is such a beautiful gift, and I suggest using it throughout the recovery process."*

I'm a big believer in the power of laughter. Sometimes you just have to try to make yourself laugh until you actually *feel* like laughing again. If you need a place to start, I suggest going on Pinterest (http://www.pinterest.com) and checking out the "Humor" category—I always find something on there that will lift my mood!

As you may remember from Chapter Two, Hilary Crist, 27, from California, said it was important for her to **do the "opposite" of negative emotions** when her "healthy voice" wasn't very strong. She said thinking this way helps her simplify decisions and make choices that are better for her. Here is an in-depth example of this portion of her process:

> *"I am at home, stressed out, tired, lonely, very unmotivated, and bored. I feel fat and ugly and want to hide indoors and isolate myself the rest of the day. I am hearing nothing but negative thoughts in my head and can see the situation developing into a full-fledged binge and purge. At this point, my healthy voice has been diminished to a mere whisper and I am almost like an observer of my body and what is unfolding. To get myself out of this self-sabotaging situation, all I have to do is the opposite of what I am feeling.*
>
> *"Feeling like lying on the couch all day alone and isolating? I get up take a shower and get dressed and leave the house. For me, this usually entails walking my*

dog. This way I am out in the sun and fresh air, taking care of something else and at the same time, taking care of myself. Feeling alone and 'stuck' in my aloneness? I call someone and become connected once again. I may write a card to my Grandma or my sister who is in Europe. If I feel worthless and feel like treating myself that way, I know I need to be gentle to myself. Maybe this means giving my feet a pedicure. I find this tip extremely effective because it does not require much thought when I am 'in the moment.'

"I know that if I am struggling, I may not always hear my healthy voice, but by doing the opposite to my emotion, I am giving my healthy self her voice back."

Hilary's process is a wonderful way to combat some of the tough feelings you'll inevitably face. Although they are a part of life, you don't have to let them derail you anymore.

Silence your inner critic. No one will ever be as critical of you as you are of yourself. When you look in the mirror in the morning and start to zero in on a new wrinkle, a pimple, or a little bit of puffiness under your eyes, it's your job to tell your inner critic to buzz off so you can focus on something you like about yourself. When you're disappointed because you didn't get the job you applied for or the "A" you worked so hard for on your exam, it's not because you're a loser or that you aren't smart enough. Once you **turn your inner critic into your inner cheerleader**, you'll be able to get the motivation you need in order to develop a better application package or figure out more effective study methods. Constant self-criticism does nothing but immobilize you further.

Try writing your own affirmation. To be perfectly honest, I always thought the idea of using affirmations sounded a little lame until I began to connect it to what I'd been learning about positive thoughts through CBT. Once I started thinking about how my feelings improve when I think more positively, the idea of using affirmations started to make a little more sense to me. To test it out for yourself, come up with a statement that is a positive representation of what you want to become or accomplish. Remember that the key to creating an effective affirmation is making it something you believe can actually happen for you. I personally would never do well with something super cheesy, like "I am the master of my universe!" Instead, I use things as simple as, "I am tough enough to get through this" or "I can accomplish anything as long as I work for it."

Keep your affirmation short and make sure it's something positive, yet still believable for you. Here are a few examples of affirmations that might work for you:

- I am happy.
- I am grateful for my life.
- My life is blessed.
- I am strong.

- I am smart enough to do anything I want.
- I can do anything, because I am persistent.
- I like myself.

Be creative when coming up with your own affirmations. What works for others might not work at all for you. You might also find that an affirmation that's worked for you in the past may do nothing at all for you today. Once you find a phrase that works for you, make sure you repeat it to yourself frequently throughout the day. Also try to really *feel* what you are saying to yourself, as you are saying it.

The difference that positive statements can make is truly amazing. One of my all-time favorite contributor stories came from Rachelle, 23, of Arizona, who shared how her mother used words to inspire her:

> *"I was having a really hard time one night and my mom came home from work early to be with me. She asked me what I wanted out of life and I started saying things that I wanted but it was hard for me to see them coming true. So she went downstairs, got a marker and started writing all over my wall. She wanted to make my wishes more visible. She started writing down whatever I said and encouraged me to do the same. After awhile, I started writing affirmations, quotes, and words of wisdom all over my wall. If I ever had a hard time I just looked at my wall and was able to see what it was I was working for."*

If you're cringing a little bit at the thought of taking a permanent marker to your walls, you can still do something similar to what Rachelle did: Just **use dry erase markers to write on your mirrors and windows**, or **write out your hopes and dreams on colorful pieces of construction paper that you can tape up** and see every day.

Pay attention when others say things that make you feel good: Did someone tell you they liked your hair this morning, or that you're a really good singer? Write down the compliments you receive, and keep them in your heart to remember on days when you start to doubt yourself.

Make a memory book. What are all of your favorite memories? Record them with as much detail as possible (visual information, scents/emotions you remember, etc.) Include any pictures or clippings you can find that relate to those experiences. Read and relive those times when you're feeling down, and remind yourself that you will have many more good experiences like them (or even better ones) in the future, just as long as you stay on track.

Give thanks and have hope. Make a list of everything you're thankful for—all of the great things you already have in your life that you want to remember when you're having a bad day. Also make a list of all of the great things you have to look forward to in your life, as long as you get healthy. Print out the lists and keep them somewhere you'll see them regularly. If you want, gather pictures that represent everything you desire and everything you already have, and post them up in your room to inspire yourself!

Play with playlists. Take some time to create different playlists of music to fit your various moods. Have a list of punk rock music for when you're angry, Christmas music for when you're feeling down and need a little cheer, or upbeat dance music when you need a boost. Building on that idea a little, my friend Laura told me she finds it helpful to identify a "theme song" that fits your personality or philosophy in life. This song can be a great mood lifter or a wonderful way to help you stay focused when you're working on a goal.

Compliment strangers and other people in your life. It's amazing how good you can feel when you brighten someone else's day! Make a special effort to compliment people for things that aren't the "standard" definition of beauty, like bright silky white hair or an outfit that could only have been devised after a thrift store visit or two.

Be assertive and **be vocal.** If someone or something is bugging you, talk about it. My husband is probably the bluntest person you'd ever meet. If I make dinner for him, I always know exactly what he thinks. He's not rude about it, but he is brutally honest. This goes well beyond dinner. And despite me being a bit of a sensitive person, I do appreciate that quality about him because I always know where he stands. There are no guessing games. If we disagree on something, we talk about it respectfully instead of just brushing it under the rug and letting it bother us.

I've taken the cue from my husband, and it's done wonders for both my emotions and my relationships. If my husband and I are making plans for the weekend and I want to spend some quality time with him, I need to actually tell him rather than waiting for him to read my mind and suggest we go on a real, official date. If I'm going out to dinner with my family and there's a new restaurant I want to try, I need to suggest it rather than us ending up going to the same places we always go. When I speak up, even if we don't always do what I've suggested, we're usually able to make some sort of compromise, and everyone is happier. If your family is trying to decide which movie to watch or where to go on vacation, speak up about what you want. People will never know how you really feel unless you tell them!

Amy Pettengill, 27, from New Hampshire said it was her tendency to hold so many things inside that triggered her eating disorder. She said that even though she talked about those things in therapy, they wouldn't get resolved without her actually communicating with others about them. She learned to be more assertive by first writing letters to people about how she felt, and then beginning to talk with some of the people she felt closer to. Nowadays, she's a lot more comfortable speaking up for herself, and has had positive results:

> *"I was at (a coffee shop) and ordered an iced latte. They gave me a hot latte, and when I informed them that they had made a mistake, the barista became angry with me and re-served me my iced latte with a negative attitude. Well, this morning when I went in, the same barista was in there, and I confronted her about her attitude yesterday and told her that I felt I was undeserving of it. She apologized, and I felt great!"*

Even though it's a little nerve-wracking at first, being assertive gets easier with practice. The trick is to use reason and speak politely. Tell the person how you're feeling and why—don't just get upset and raise your voice without fully explaining things to them. Also make sure that you are ready and willing to listen to and try to understand their perspective as well—after all, there may be pieces of the puzzle that you don't already know about.

Let go of guilt and the pressure you put on yourself to be the perfect person for everyone around you. It's not your job to make sure your friends and family are happy at all times; it's theirs. I'm not telling you to go out there and be a butthead to everyone, but you'll never be happy if you're always putting yourself last. If you're a religious person, **remember that God doesn't expect you to be perfect either.** You might mess up sometimes, but you can fix it. Living a good life is a constant process, just like recovery. **Don't forget to take care of yourself throughout your quest to help others,** because God also wants you to be happy. **Take some time for yourself every day, to relax and do things that make you feel good** (Remember Chapter Three?). If you're anything like me, you're a much better, nicer person when you're happy!

Kelly Michaels, 39, from Minnesota, said it helped her to **keep a "God Box":** a box where she could put all of the worries she wrote down on slips of paper. She said, "Once you put (your worries) into the box, you are handing your problems over to God to take care of. Doing something physical like that helps more than just thinking it."

Focus on the present and future more than on the past. Dwelling on mistakes you've made or negative things that have happened is a surefire way to make you feel depressed or irritated. **Pay attention to all of the positive things you have in your life right now, and what you can do at this moment to create a healthier, happier future.** You can't change the past, but you can learn from it.

Stay in the moment, and keep your eyes open. There's an amazing amount of beauty in the world around you. Jenni, 24, from Texas, shared a journal excerpt in which she reflected on how detached she was in her own life:

> *"The only time I was present today was at breakfast because it's my favorite*

meal, though I was multitasking and reading the paper. While walking Deuce (my dog) I was thinking about getting tan. I was somewhere else while I was driving. At my meeting I was thinking about my massage. During my massage I was thinking about going shopping and how fat my legs must've looked and what to journal about and how I didn't want to eat...and how I wasn't present. At the restaurant I was eager to get home. At home I wanted to be back at the restaurant. Did I just waste the whole day wanting to be somewhere else?"

If you want to learn to live in the moment more, **try removing all of the clocks from your house for one day.** Remember to also put your watch away. Have a friend or family member let you know when it's time for a meal or snack, and then follow what's on your meal plan. You might also want to have them tell you when it's close to your bedtime, so you don't end up going to sleep at 4 a.m. if you have somewhere to be the next day. Other than that, the day's activities are up to you! Have a list of potential activities ready, and then just do whatever you feel like doing, for however long you feel like doing it. Your job is to have fun and focus on each instant as it comes, rather than thinking about what you will be doing later.

Deb K., 43, from North Carolina, said it wasn't until she learned to manage her emotions and be present in each moment that she was able to "recover" her children emotionally:

"I had always cared for them physically, until in my eating disorder I drove myself down to exhaustion and weakness and had to be hospitalized. Then my husband or mother or mother-in-law had to take over. Over and over again I created this cycle. And then, even when I was home I was present physically, but as soon as stress and tension hit (and there's none of that raising six children, is there?), I would go somewhere in my head—somewhere they couldn't go. Of course they didn't understand, but they could feel it when I 'wasn't there.' But as I regained physical, emotional, and spiritual health in recovery, I found myself able and eager to look each one of them in the eyes as they shared the stories of their precious days with me. They could see the attentiveness and understanding in my eyes, and they gobbled it up. No more, 'Mommy look at me,' with their little hands around my cheeks guiding my face to look at them. No more, 'Mommy, are you sleeping again?' I was right there with them."

It's essential to stay connected with others. No matter how much you might sometimes feel like curling up in a little ball and isolating yourself from the world, it really is your positive relationships with others that will keep you emotionally healthy. Spending time with other people will help you get your mind off of some of your worries, especially if you're talking about something else or doing something you enjoy. See Chapter Five for more.

Keep your heart and mind open. Try not to get upset if things don't always go exactly how you think they should. Black and white aren't the only colors in your crayon box, and things can't often be seen as simply "right" or "wrong." If you're like me, you might remember a time when you were a kid and thought everything your parents said was the absolute only truth. However, no matter how smart your parents are, the world is full of different people, different perspectives, and different answers. There are countless numbers of recipes you can use to make a chocolate cake (or you can make Funfetti instead, like I would!). You can take several different routes to get to a single place.

One of the most significant things I've learned is that for me personally, most of the really intense, difficult feelings I have, come when I start to feel that lack of control over certain things in my life. Like most people, when it seems like nothing is going my way, I might start to feel frazzled, depressed, or even kind of angry. I've learned that when this happens I usually have to do something physical for a little while, but then just take some really deep breaths and relax: I have to engage a calmer state of mind and reframe my thoughts, reminding myself that all of the things in my life don't have to fit into perfect little boxes that are kept in a perfect little order. I've often found that when things don't exactly go the way I want them to, the outcomes turn out to be even better! There is a lot of beauty and excitement to be found in a world that you *can't* control, and you'll be a lot happier once you learn to embrace and explore it.

Listen to yourself, trust yourself, and if you're a spiritual person like me, **trust in God's plan for you.** As much as I hate to admit it, I've learned that I *don't* really know what's best for me all the time. However, even if I can't control the exact direction my life will go in, I can listen to what's in my heart a little more. For me, it's God's voice, telling me to be patient and trust that what I need will come to me when the time is right. It wasn't until I finally started trusting God that I was able to more easily endure all the inevitable little bumps in my life, knowing that as long as I just kept moving forward, everything would fall into its right place in the end. In the past when I tried to rush into a relationship, I ended up with both a broken heart and a broken life. When I finally decided to place my life wholly in God's hands, it wasn't very long before I met Todd, the love of my life. I won't fib and say that my life is always easy and perfect now (whose is?), but I can say that there is true joy and peace in my heart now.

Find healthier things than your weight to "control." Whenever I used to start to feel a little bit overwhelmed by some of the random things in my life, my first instinct was always to step on the scale, so I could pretend I was in control of something (sound familiar?). Obviously, this is one little habit that needs to go (see Chapter Eight)! The important thing to remember is that even though it is just about impossible to completely control anything in your life, you *are* in complete control of how you *respond* to whatever happens to you. You also can make healthy routines and good decisions that will help you at least *direct* your life down a positive path. If you haven't already, start meeting regularly with a counselor or coach to chart some life goals, or begin working your way through some of the activities in Chapter Three.

Embrace your new emotional experience. Rachael (who asked not to share her age because she hates numbers!), from New York, is an example of how much richer life can be when it's filled with true feeling. She said she was surprised by how much she actually enjoys her emotions now: "It took me almost two years to be able to feel as deeply as I do, and it provides a depth to life that I would never want to live without."

Remember that you are loved. Regardless of how you feel about yourself sometimes, there are people in your life whose worlds are much brighter because of you. No matter what you've done in the past, or how many times you have failed at something, you still deserve to be happy and live a good life. From a religious perspective, God doesn't ever give up on you or stop loving you, even if you're not always a "perfect" person. Every day is a new opportunity to do better, and to become the kind of person you truly desire to be.

Find a way to love yourself. Kelly Michaels, 39, from Minnesota learned to love herself after having her daughter, who she knew would grow up watching her. She began healing her childhood wounds by striving to love herself in the same way that she would love a child: "I have a baby photo of me in my bathroom and I say hi to 'the baby' every morning. Funny and weird concept, but it has worked wonderfully for learning to be gentle to myself in a way that I never could before."

Discover true inner peace. Have you ever chased after something (a relationship, some sort of success, money, or other material good), only to find that as soon as you attained it, you didn't feel any happier or more satisfied than when you began? Although I don't remember where it came from specifically, I once read somewhere that the "empty" feeling you have inside of you at times may actually be a longing for God. Even though you may have your own spiritual beliefs, the idea is one that really resonated with me. It made sense to me that perhaps that strange feeling of always desiring…*something*…could be attributed to me actually feeling a little bit disconnected with God. I learned that the times in my life when I thought I needed a boyfriend or new clothes or a different body to be happy, were really times when I needed to feel closer to God. Now **when I start to feel something negative stirring up inside me, I make time for some good conversation with God:** I talk to Him about how I'm feeling, ask questions about whatever it is I'm having trouble dealing with or understanding, and open my heart for direction. I always feel much more relaxed when I'm finished. Give it a try yourself, or **if you're not a religious person, try regularly setting aside some time for meditation**

or yoga. Both can be great ways for you to get centered and find your own answers from within yourself.

What if, despite all your best efforts, you're still having a lot of trouble dealing with your emotions? Is something like medication the answer, or should you keep trying to get better without it? If you do choose to utilize medication, what are some guidelines for incorporating it into your recovery plan?

There's no single answer to any of those questions, because everyone is unique. The best answer is that you should talk to your physician and therapist to see what's right for you. Until then, here's what I've learned about medication's role in recovery:

Where Does Medication Fit In?

Before going on any medication, it's important to **know the difference between normal emotions (like sadness or nervousness) and emotional extremes (such as depression or chronic anxiety).** No amount of medication (or counseling for that matter) will ever completely take away every bit of sadness or fear from your life, because some of those feelings will just always naturally occur. Emotions are part of the richness of the human experience: After all, how would you ever know what genuine happiness felt like if you had never been sad?

True depression and anxiety, however, are very different from everyday emotions: Anxiety and depression last longer than a few moments or a few days. The nervousness or sadness that go along with them may not seem to have a specific reason. They are also severe enough to the point where they may interfere with your ability to carry on with your normal life. If you are depressed, you may not ever feel like getting out of bed in the morning, no matter how much you've slept. If you have anxiety, you may not want to leave your house, even if you've been feeling very lonely lately and some friends have invited you over for a movie. For either, you may feel as though you are constantly ill (stomachaches, headaches, dizziness, etc.), even if a physician's examination determines you to be physically healthy.

If you are experiencing emotional distress that you believe may be inhibiting your ability to live your life, get an evaluation from your counselor, therapist, or physician. Then, depending on your results you may want to talk with them about your medication options.

Medication is a personal choice. I don't use it, because I've done a lot of learning about both myself and my thought patterns, to the point where I'm now able to regulate my emotions pretty well. No matter what happens to me in my daily life, I know how to positively structure my thoughts so that I'm able to stay relatively optimistic. However, I have friends and family members who have said that medication has made a world of difference in their lives. For some, it helps them think more clearly or gives them the physical or mental boost they need to help them make healthy changes. The medication people take for their emotions can be likened to those taken by people with other conditions: If they might help alleviate your symptoms and improve your daily life to the point where you are able to learn the skills you need to manage your emotions more easily, they are worth being considered.

If you do decide to try medication, remember that you might need to try different types and dosages before you find what works best for you. Everyone is unique, and you might not find the perfect combination right away. That's why it's so important to keep a good relationship with both your physician and your counselor or therapist, so they can help you monitor how the medication is affecting you both physically and emotionally. **Be proactive in educating yourself about different medication options,** so you can visit with your physician and counselor about what you think might be most helpful for you. Also **be honest with your therapist or physician if you think something isn't working for you.** If you don't start feeling more like "you" after a few weeks (or however long your physician tells you it may take), it's probably time to reevaluate your plan.

If you use medication, know that **it's only part of the process:** You will still need to learn to understand and deal with your emotions in a healthy way. You'll also need to take care of yourself physically—after all, it's hard to feel good inside when your body is weak or hurting! Make sure you're getting enough sleep and a *healthy* amount of exercise. Also keep in mind that because of the effects malnutrition has on your emotions, **even with medication you might not notice any improvement until you reach a healthy weight.** I noticed a drastic difference in myself once I began eating right, even without medication: I had more energy, could think more clearly, and wasn't constantly restricting myself. It only makes sense that my mood was better.

Finally, know that **for many people, medication isn't a permanent solution.** It is often thought of as a "bridge" for people as they learn how to understand and respond to their own emotional tendencies. Many people are able to taper off their medication once they get to that point.

Be honest with yourself about what might be best for you: Although it took a lot of work and self-awareness on my part, I was able to completely transform my way of thinking and feeling, without medication. I am still an anxious person sometimes, but I've recognized that it's actually a part of my personality, and I don't let it go to extremes anymore. Like most people, I do still feel sad from time to time, but it usually doesn't last for very long and I'm able to manage it in a healthy way.

Stay conscious of your feelings. Even if they're not always easy, they *are* only temporary, and they in themselves can't hurt you or stop you from doing anything you want to do! Pay attention if you start to notice yourself gritting your teeth or balling your hands up into fists. Concentrate on relaxing your muscles, calming your mind, and allowing yourself to release some of that tension. Flood your mind with good thoughts so you can wash away the bad ones. If you're anxious, go for a walk in the fresh air or do something with your hands, like playing with modeling clay or knitting. If you're depressed, call up someone you love for a chat, or even better, ask them to meet up with you somewhere so you can reconnect.

Whether you believe it or not, **you really can regain control of your emotions.** Humans have an amazing ability to adapt: If you're taking care of yourself both inside and out, you'll be able to develop healthier responses and transform your whole outlook on life.

For me personally, the biggest difference in my emotional state today versus a few years ago is that I now have a trust in both God and in myself that I never had before. I had to go through a huge learning process, but I know now that despite experiencing both an eating disorder and a traumatic relationship, I *am* okay both physically and emotionally, and I will be able to handle anything that comes my way. I've learned to trust that there is a plan for my life that will continue to unfold as it is meant to unfold.

The same is true for you: From this day on, stop futilely trying to control your life—just live it, and savor the journey!

Now, here are this chapter's journal questions, followed by the family and Q & A sections:

Journal Questions

1. Write about any strong emotions you experience: What thoughts preceded those emotions? How did those thoughts influence your emotions? If the emotions are negative, how can you upcycle your thoughts to create a more positive feeling?

2. What are all of the good things that happened to you today (List as many as possible!)? What are you grateful for in your life today?

3. What are some of the negative thoughts you have sometimes? What do those thoughts tell you that convince you to believe them? What kinds of things can you say to fight back against those negative thoughts?

Tips for Friends & Family

Try not to take things personally.

Many parts of recovery are just downright hard: Those who are recovering are making changes they don't always want to make, without always knowing how to deal with some of their emotions.

No matter how emotional or angry your loved one might seem at times, it likely isn't a reflection on their feelings for you. They are going through some difficult things, but they really do love you. Meg, 16, from Nottingham, England, said that despite some tough moments, her mother never forgot that Meg cared about her:

> *"Understand the sufferer isn't in control 100% of the time, and it's kind of a Dr. Jekyl and Mr. Hyde thing. My mum refers to me as Meg A (my anorexic behaviors) and Meg B (her daughter). She knows Meg B loves her even if Meg A will get mad because she is making her eat more."*

Let me feel my feelings.

Even if some of your loved one's feelings may not seem to make sense, he or she needs to feel a sense of validation. Emotions are kind of like food cravings, in that you have to respond to them *before* they get out of hand. Your loved one will also be more likely to keep talking to you if he or she knows you are really listening.

Consider taking part in counseling yourself.

Getting involved in family sessions will help you better understand what your loved one is going through and how you can help him or her. Allie, 23, from Pennsylvania said that family therapy can have a significant impact on a loved one's recovery:

> *"I would definitely suggest attending some family therapy sessions, but after the person suffering from the disorder has had several of their own with that same therapist. It's really positive and incredibly important for the person struggling with an eating disorder to see their family's support…"*

Also make sure you have someone you can talk to about your own feelings and challenges. This person should be someone who understands some of the specific things you're dealing with. Allie, 23, from Pennsylvania said that it was "amazing" to know that while she was away at college, her mother was attending an eating disorder-specific group so she could not only help herself, but become an even better support for her daughter.

Take care of yourself.

Remember to take time to do things that calm you and take your mind off of your worries. Get some healthy exercise and spend time with friends *without* talking about your loved one's eating disorder. Get plenty of sleep and eat a balanced diet. Doing these things will allow you to not only be a stronger support for your loved one, but also a healthy example.

Be patient.

Recovery won't happen overnight. Suzanne Yerdon Lewandowski, 55, from Massachusetts pointed out the fact that at the beginning of recovery, everything feels "wrong" and "foreign" because "one's inner being is at war with itself." She compared it to trying to put together a jigsaw puzzle:

> *"...many pieces need to be tried when cultivating new intellectual, physical, relational, and spiritual aspects of the person. It may take many tries before the first pieces fit. Relapse may be the result of a piece that does not work. The sufferer must keep trying, changing, evolving. Many pieces are needed before the recovery picture fills in, and you can look back and see significant progress. Slowly, the tentacles will lose their hold as health, strength, and purpose return. As the loved one, your challenge is to encourage motivation and provide hope."*

Julia, 23, from Worcestershire, England said that although it can be challenging to support someone who feels trapped between their eating disorder and recovery, it is possible:

> *"They may accept or reject other people's concerns. It's extremely frustrating, but try not to get angry if they don't seem to 'hear' what you're saying. Eating issues are hugely complex and confusing, so a sufferer's reactions do not necessarily reflect their feelings. They may feel trapped and torn between taking the steps towards recovery, or ignoring the possibility of change and stubbornly staying put. This must be hurtful for those on the outside looking in, and supporting that person is tricky, but possible. Just try not to let your own anxieties affect them."*

Ashley Devitt, 18, from Florida added that it's important to not rush your loved one through their process or ever give up on them, "because if you do not have faith in the one you love, why should he or she have faith in themselves?"

Believe.

Trust that your loved one will get better as long as you continue to support and encourage them. Julia, 23, from Worcestershire, England added that it is only now that she has recovered that she can understand how distressing it must have been for her friends and family to see her struggling with her disorder:

> *"At my very worst, I felt both furious and immensely guilty towards my parents for their being so stressed about my condition, but for years I felt helpless to change my ways. Their love for me despite my intolerable behaviors, and their astounding faith in my pending recovery, meant I was lucky enough to have a reliable source of support that helped me take the courage to pursue recovery. So many of the positive changes in my life over the last few years were due to their sheer perseverance and belief in me that I could and would get better."*

Julia's story of transformation isn't unique. Below is a journal excerpt from Ashley Devitt on how her relationship with her family has changed throughout her recovery:

July 22, 2007

> *I saw my mom cry today. I think it hurt me more than it hurt her. I didn't know if I should stay around and comfort her or hide myself from the reality of it all. I hate this. I hate to see my mom cry. And I hate that I'm the reason for her tears. Not only do I hate that I have done the things I've done, but I hate even more that I continue to do the things I do. I hate that I have to go around hurting everyone who loves me, when the only person I really want to hurt is myself. I don't know why my family still cares for me. After all that I've done, I don't understand why they love me. I've betrayed them, lied to them, broken their hearts, and yet they still support me. I guess they're able to see the innocent girl beneath the villain, even though I have yet to see her.*

March 14, 2009

> *Today I was asked by my school's guidance counselor to speak to a young group of girls about the importance of being healthy. It didn't really hit me until now, but I have really come a long way since the depths of my eating disorder. Mrs. H., who has been my guidance counselor throughout my struggles and my journey toward recovery, asked me how I did it. I've never really thought about that before. Recovery seemed to happen so gradually. Yet, now that I've come so far along, it seems almost surreal—it feels like just yesterday that I was yelling and screaming at anyone who dared put food in front of me.*

But in reality, that was so long ago. That got me to thinking…I have put my family through hell, yet they have always supported me. I'm not sure why, but I'm really fortunate. Even when I lost faith in myself, my family never did. Even when I wanted to die, my family wanted me to live–despite the fact that I could be a real pain. And looking back, I am so glad that they did. I've always wanted to thank them for their unconditional love, but I've never found a way. But something tells me that they know how much I appreciate it. It's like that unspoken language between us. Every time they see me smile, I think they know that I'm thankful to be here. Maybe someday I'll be able to find the words to tell them how grateful I am. But for now, I think my actions speak for themselves.

Questions Friends & Family Should Ask

1. What would you like me to know about you and how you really feel?
2. What was the best thing that happened to you today?
3. What's something that happened that wasn't so great? What's something positive we can take or learn from that?

Journal Questions for Friends & Family

1. How am I feeling throughout my loved one's recovery?
2. How can I get support for myself?
3. What are some other things I can do to take care of myself?

Q & A with Carolyn Costin, MFT, M.ED, and Keesha Broome, M.A., MFT

Q: How do I find a good therapist? How do I know if my relationship with my therapist is working for me?

A: A therapist's services are something you are consuming so you should treat it as any other important purchase—shop around. Ask questions about the therapist's experience, technique, expertise. Trust your instinct. If you feel comfortable with a particular therapist, that can be as important—if not more—than their experience. Find someone with whom you feel safe to talk. Make a list of important qualities and then find the therapist who meets these.

Q: Should I go on medication?

A: It is often difficult to discern whether or not the symptoms you are experiencing warrant medication or will be healed by eliminating behaviors. This question is best addressed by a psychiatrist, with a specialty in eating disorders, who can prescribe and manage medication. If you do not have a psychiatrist, your therapist or primary care physician should be able to refer you to one.

Often, individuals with eating disorders do not like to take medication. There can be an overwhelming fear of the potential side effects or a belief that taking medication will negatively alter personality. It is important to get educated by a physician or nurse about what specific medications do and how they can be helpful to you. We have seen many people find such relief from obsessive thoughts, ritualistic behavior, severe depression, and intolerable anxiety by finding the proper medication.

It is also important to note that nutritional rehabilitation should take place before going on medication. You want to make sure that, for example, you are not medicating a depression that would lift with regular eating and weight restoration.

5 Your Dinner Companions: Recreating relationships

"Keep love in your heart. A life without it is like a sunless garden when the flowers are dead. The consciousness of loving and being loved brings a warmth and richness to life that nothing else can bring."

–Oscar Wilde

Despite everything you read in Chapter Three about my lack of a childhood social life, I wasn't a complete loner. I did have a best friend—even if she did have thick pink glasses and the nickname "Crybaby," and even if she did earn her grade-school notoriety by throwing up all over our teacher's desk in the first grade. She had a heart of gold, and I always knew she cared. I think more people should have friends with thick pink glasses.

I also had my first boyfriend in kindergarten. I still remember how he stopped in front of my desk on Valentine's Day, and then shyly handed me a brown paper bag. Inside the bag was a little red heart-shaped box of five chocolates, with a big red polyester rose attached to the top. My kindergarten boyfriend would stand behind me in line at the water fountain and we would pretend to eat the plastic fruit on my bracelet (quite romantic). At recess he chased me around, and I would always run away, because A) I was shy, and B) I wasn't sure if I really liked him in "that way." After awhile, he stopped chasing me. He moved away for a couple of years, and came back for awhile in 3rd grade. We didn't talk about the chocolates he had given me, or any of our playground escapades. We didn't talk at all—I think talking about that unrequited love would probably have been a little awkward for both of us.

The first boy I liked who wasn't my kindergarten boyfriend was one I met in first grade. I liked him simply and solely because he had spiky hair. It's actually a little ironic, because I was always a little jealous of the fact that my own hair was too long for me to be able to spike it. Regardless, the spiky-haired boy never noticed me—and neither did a lot of the boys I liked while growing up. It became a common theme for me: The boys who were interested in me could never catch me. The boys with spiky hair apparently just had poor vision (and mental capacities).

By the time I got to college, I thought it was probably a little weird that I'd never had a serious boyfriend. I didn't think the guy I exchanged long, obnoxious letters with and drove aimlessly around parking lots with for two weeks really counted, although we did have a lot of fun together. Neither did the guy I often shared mini candy bars with and dated off and on, but could never look directly at because of my friend's constant comments about his shaggy eyebrows (Yes—extraordinarily shallow of me, I am aware. And yes, she probably *was* just jealous, either of our relationship or the fact that she was not involved in the candy bar-sharing).

When I first got to college, I was very lonely. I missed my family, and my new atmosphere most certainly hadn't transformed me into an extrovert overnight. I did meet someone my first day at college—the best friend of a guy who had a crush on my roommate. Needless to say, both guys were over at our room every single night. He and I had absolutely nothing in common beyond the fact that he was also missing his family, and looking for a relationship. We started dating officially within just a couple of weeks. Superficially-speaking, it was the perfect combination: He was looking for someone pretty to validate him, and I thought that dating him—a football player at my new school—would not only give me some company on lonely nights, but also the social status I had always felt to be lacking in high school.

Throughout the first few months of our relationship, it was clear enough to me that he didn't seem to respect me: He flirted with other girls in front of me. He didn't often call when he said he would. He was possessive and always seemed to have his hands on me—I couldn't even stand up straight when we walked together because of how restrictively he always wrapped his arm over my shoulders. Physically, he pushed me to do things I really didn't want to do, and that made me feel horrible afterward.

After five months, I broke up with him. I wrote him a long, honest letter, finally telling him about all of the things that bothered me about our relationship. I told him he didn't respect me or treat me the way he should. I said all of the things I had always been too afraid to say in person. After he'd had a chance to read the letter, we talked on the phone for a really long time. In that phone conversation, as was typical of our relationship, we avoided really talking about anything in the letter. Despite that, I was amazed by how easily we suddenly seemed to be able to talk to each other about all kinds of other random subjects. It was like I was talking to a totally different person.

No matter how they happen, breakups are hard (duh). About a week and a half after I gave my old boyfriend that letter, I saw him in a gym on our campus, all alone. I wasn't sure if he had seen me or not. He had just kept walking. I began thinking again about our last phone conversation, and how we had actually *talked* to each other for once. As ridiculous as it sounds, I also felt a little bad for him. Despite how poorly he had treated me, I'd spent so much time with him over those months that I actually did care about him. I felt guilty for breaking up with him, when I knew how much he already was hurting from being away from his family. When I asked my suitemate what she thought I should do, she said, "Honestly? I see you guys getting back together."

I started to think that maybe I needed to give him a second chance. I sent him a long email, and then called him and told him to read it.

This time, we stayed together for five years. I hate to admit the fact that there were plenty of times throughout those five years when I really, really thought I could be making a mistake by being with him. I didn't really like his personality, and he didn't get along with my family very well. He had a short fuse, and threatened to physically harm my sister and her boyfriend-now-husband (who is one of the sweetest, calmest people I've ever met) if they ever did anything that sparked his anger. He frequently lied to me when he did things he knew I wouldn't like. But even with all of this going on, a scared little voice inside me told me I couldn't leave him. I felt morally bound to him because of our physical and emotional history together. Beyond that, from the very first weeks of our relationship he had often made references to "our kids" that we would have together someday. I allowed his staunch belief in our future—our destiny!—together, to convince me to ignore all of my own stark doubts.

Even if I hadn't cared about any of that, he was my sole "support system" while I was away from my family. I was afraid I would never find anyone else (boyfriend *or* friend) if I left. All of my friends disappeared soon after I started dating him, and at the end of the day, I didn't think I could survive on my own. It didn't matter if people said I was pretty, or smart, or whatever—leaving was a risk I didn't want to take.

A couple of years into the relationship, I sort of stopped eating. I was in the midst of trying to recover from bulimia, and I didn't remember how to eat like a normal person. For me at that time, under-eating offered me not only a false sense of control over my diet and my life, but also a means of attempting to tell my boyfriend how distraught I was about so many aspects of our relationship. Whenever I ate dinner with him, I wondered if he'd notice something was wrong when he saw all of the untouched food on my plate, and ask me to start talking. I wished I knew how to bring up those conversations myself, in a way that he would actually respond to, but I didn't know how and I was afraid to try. So I kept quiet, and let my slowly shrinking body do its own talking.

I don't know if he ever really understood all the reasons behind the weight I lost over the next couple of years; I don't think I even did for a very long time afterward. I do know that he hated it. As much as he was able to control and shape my behavior in so many other areas, he was never able to make me eat.

It would have been hard to leave that relationship while I was still in college. I would have had to spend a fair amount of time walking across campus by myself, thinking about what a "loser" I was. I would have had to spend some evenings alone in my depressing, white brick jail cell of a dorm room. There probably would have been nights when I didn't sleep at all because of my anxiety. But things get harder the longer you wait.

I wish I could say I chose to leave him and that relationship, but I didn't; I was planning on staying with him forever. It didn't matter that I thought I could do better—that I *deserved* better—or that he never seemed to "get" me or my sense of humor. I tried not to think about the fact that we never enjoyed just talking to each other, and that he was so *not* the kind of person I'd always envisioned myself being with when I was younger.

The last couple of years we spent together were not so great for either of us. He sat in the dark playing video games for most of the day while I was at work, and even at night after I'd gone to bed. No matter how much he always denied that anything was wrong, he was just as unhappy with his life as I was with mine.

In the last year of our relationship, the only talking we really did was when we argued. Still, nothing I said ever seemed to really permeate him; his eyes were often cold, hard, and empty, kind of like those on a dead fish. He told me I was crazy when I tried to tell him how I felt about us, or life, or myself. He told me I was too "messed up" from my eating disorder to be thinking clearly about anything at all. He said my eating disorder and I were the cause of all of the problems in our relationship. To him, it was unreasonable for me to be bothered by any of his behaviors. He said my emotions were all wrong, and that I just needed to be sent away somewhere to be "fixed."

It was after he said those kinds of things that I began to talk about leaving. I don't think either of us ever really believed I would actually do it. He insisted that emotionally I couldn't survive without him, and that physically, I needed him to protect me. He told me I would never be able to make friends without him, because in his mind, I didn't know how to talk to people.

He started leaving our apartment to go sit in his truck when he received phone calls, so I wouldn't be able to hear what he was saying. He started lying to me more, and becoming even angrier at the most unpredictable moments. Sometimes during our arguments he would pick me up and shake me, or hold me down on the floor so I couldn't move while he yelled at me. It was hard for me to believe that despite all my childhood dreams of a fairytale romance, I was part of the couple in our apartment building who were known for always screaming at each other.

In time, although I wasn't really sure why, I began to notice myself feeling afraid when I was around him, like I had to be careful about everything I said or did. I tried to push those feelings out of my mind. I knew we were having some problems, but it seemed wrong of me to be afraid of the very person who was supposed to love me like no one else.

Reality set in a little more for me on a weekend trip we took to a nearby town to celebrate one of our anniversaries. We had stopped at a shopping mall for a little bit, and he had become angry about something, although I honestly don't remember what it was. I do remember feeling a little shocked, because whatever it was had seemed rather trivial to me. That day, in the middle of the food court, he placed both of his hands on my shoulders and shook me as he yelled at me. I squeezed back my tears and pleaded with him to stop, aware of all of the curious and stunned eyes that were on us.

When he was finished yelling, we each went to separate lines to get something to eat. A woman in line next to me asked me if he was my boyfriend. I shook my head and stared down at my feet, ashamed. How could I tell her that *that* person was the one I thought I had to spend the rest of my life with? The woman was silent for a moment before saying her final words to me: "If he was, I wouldn't stay with him."

I knew she was right. But it was another 10 months until I took her advice.

In the last few weeks of our relationship, I was having panic attacks almost daily, and I was hardly sleeping anymore. It was difficult for me to go to work because I was terrified I might pass out from all of the emotional distress and exhaustion, right there in front of my bosses. I got a prescription for medication to use during panic attacks, although it didn't really help. I started to think I really *was* going crazy, just like *he* so often said I was. I began to feel very uncomfortable every time I was in a public place; I was terrified that I might just have a nervous breakdown sometime when I was out in front of others, and unable to escape their stares.

As I mentioned in Chapter One, my mom picked me up from work on what ended up being my last day there. Even though she lives about 100 miles away, she had been in town for a conference. On that day, I had had such a bad panic attack that I couldn't even pretend to hide it from my bosses. I was lying on the floor, pale and shivering uncontrollably, with my feet up on my desk and my coat covering me. My bosses asked me if they needed to take me to the doctor. I told them that my mom was on her way. It was in my apartment building's parking lot that day, after my mother had picked me up from work, that I looked at her from across the car and asked her if I was going crazy.

In the moments after that question, we went up the stairs to my apartment together because she was worried about me. She was on the phone with my dad, telling him that she was going to be home a little late, when we entered the apartment. My dad told me later that over the phone, he heard my ex begin to scream at me as I walked in, and that the screaming had seemed to stop when he saw that I wasn't alone. I don't remember that. There are a lot of things from that time in my life that I have trouble remembering. I guess there are just some memories that are best left forgotten.

It took me going to an abused adult advocacy agency with my mom before I really started to believe that things in my relationship were not just bad—they were actually quite messed up. I still remember the woman at the agency looking across her desk at me and saying, "I know you think it'd be hard to leave right now, but what's it going to be like when you're back here in my office in ten years?"

I knew I had put things off long enough. I already felt like I was falling apart. I didn't want to think about how things would be in ten more years. The woman at the office advised me not to go back, but to go home with my mom. She said my parents could go back to my apartment sometime within the next week to get my clothes, and that when they did, they could give him a letter from me that said we could possibly reunite in the future, if he agreed to go through a treatment program. She did warn me that sometimes when people go through the programs, they don't really make the changes they need to make—they just learn how to cover things up better.

That was the day I knew *I* finally had to make the changes I had always been too afraid to make before: I had to get out of the destructive relationship that had always felt so deceptively "safe" and comfortable, and start developing my own backbone. I had to trust myself, be independent, and face my fears so that I could actually conquer them. **I had to start actively dealing with all of my problems and worries, instead of trying to cover them up with my eating disorder.** I had to trust that God would help me get wherever it was I needed to be, instead of trying to control everything myself, and ending up somewhere completely wrong.

The night before I left everything—my ex, my home, and even my job—there were clouds in the sky like I had never seen in my life—and have never seen since. They were bright, interconnected clouds that ran across the entire evening sky like soft, pillowy scales on a giant ethereal sea creature. I felt my heart lift when I saw those clouds; it was like a message from God that I was going to be all right.

After I left, I did still feel a little bit crazy for awhile. I literally felt like my whole world had crashed down and shattered all around me in tiny, jagged little pieces. I thought I had just killed any chance I'd had at someday having a real family of my own. I was embarrassed by the fact that I was living with my parents again. I was suffering so much psychologically that I was afraid I would never be capable of holding any sort of real job again. I wasn't even sure I'd be able to be in public places for very long without panic starting to take over.

In those first days, I comforted myself with thoughts that maybe things with my ex could still work out. Maybe, like in the letter I was writing to him, he would be receptive to the idea of going to a treatment program. Maybe he would actually do the other things I was writing in the letter too, like spend some time with me to just listen and learn to talk to me.

My parents told me that when they went back to our apartment to get some of my clothes out and give him the letter, he just crumpled the letter up and threw it back at them. He played with his rifles on the living room floor while they gathered my clothes.

I never saw him again. It was better that way. I had been so emotionally connected to him for so long that I was afraid if I did see him, I might want to go back. That's the funny thing about relationships. Sometimes it doesn't matter how horribly someone treats you, or how unhappy you are together—you still have a strong bond for awhile, even if it is a sick and twisted one. Bad relationships are very much like eating disorders.

Because I never saw him again, I also healed a lot more quickly: Despite all of my fears, it only took a couple of months before I felt ready to get another job, and even get an apartment of my own. As much as I love my parents, I wanted to move on with my life. Every day was hard; I had to get used to spending a lot more time alone. I still struggled with thoughts that I was going to spend my whole life by myself. On my hardest nights, I wrote letters reminding myself to have faith and remember all of the little ways God had taken care of me throughout all the tumult of the previous months: My mom being in town when I needed her that terrifying day at work. My mom and sister both being home with me during the first couple of difficult months, because everything had happened while they were on summer vacation. Me eventually finding a cozy, adorable apartment—*my* apartment—in a building that just so happened to be owned by one of my favorite professors from college. The apartment was also directly across the street from two very nice girls I had always liked but never hung out with while in college. Suddenly, I had friends.

As I began making more of an effort to take care of myself physically, many of my fears began to lessen. **Once my body had the nutrition and rest it needed, I actually felt stronger, and more confident and capable.** I fought back my old worries about my body somehow being responsible for whether or not people liked me; I reminded myself that anyone who was really worth my time—friend or boyfriend—would find my kindness, genuineness, and sense of humor to be much more of a reason to spend time with me than the size of my jeans. I got along with people much better once my eating improved, too: My mind became clear and I was able to get actively involved in conversations and make people laugh, instead of always ruminating on my last meal or my next workout.

Over the next year, I actually dated a lot. I wanted to do what I had never really gotten the chance to do in high school or college—get to know all kinds of different guys. I dated a lot of nice guys. I dated guys who were funny, guys who had good jobs, and guys who always went to church. But I never went out with any of them for more than two dates, because none of them were quite what I was looking for. I wanted to be with someone who really understood me, and who not only made me laugh, but also inspired me and challenged me. I wanted someone I could talk with for hours, and not even realize how much time had passed. I needed someone who respected me, never lied to me, and truly, honestly, *loved* me. I never broke my "two date" rule for any of those guys who weren't quite "it" for me; I knew that getting attached to any of them would only keep me from finally meeting the one who *would* be able to fill that special place in my heart.

If you know me, don't be surprised if I've given you the vague, generic story of how I met my husband. The story goes something like this: "Well, both of us have relatives who live in Who-ville (not really the name of the town, but you get the point), and his grandma even always sat right behind my brother and his family in church every weekend." I don't really consider it a lie because it is all true—there's just a little more to the story.

Since I'm clearly not hiding anything in this book, the whole, precise truth is that we met online. Now, I don't consider myself a walking advertisement for internet dating: I think if you really are able to meet someone while you're picking out oranges at the grocery store, it can make a really great story. But when you're looking for some very specific qualities in a person, like I was, something like online dating only makes sense. It's unmatched in its efficiency: Similar political views? Check. Same religious beliefs? Check. Deep-seated aversion to circus clowns? Double check—you won't ever have to worry about this guy casually mentioning on your third date that he spends his weekends wearing white paint and frequenting children's birthday parties.

Before I met Todd, I was almost as burnt out of the whole online dating scene as I was of the real-world kind. Plenty of the guys on there seemed nice enough, but I knew they just weren't for me. My parents used to roll their eyes at me because I would come home depressed sometimes, expressing my anguish over the fact that I was never going to meet anyone. They'd say something like, "Justine—you just went on two dates this week. You met another guy at the gym, and we heard you talking to someone else on the phone earlier. You're meeting people all the time." They warned me that I was maybe being a little too picky—but could you blame me? After what I'd gone through, I knew I didn't want to be with somebody just to be with *somebody*. Life is too short, and I loved having my own life back too much to just share all of it with someone whose soul didn't match mine. My little sister, her boyfriend, and I all half-jokingly agreed that if I never did find anyone I wanted to be with, I would just move in with them after they got married, and help them take care of their kids. They promised me that no matter what, I really never would be all "alone."

Today, I'm far from alone. I'm still really close to my family, and I have *real* friends who would never even think about prank calling me during any of their slumber parties (not to mention the fact that I'd actually be *invited* to those parties in the first place). Once I finally began surrounding myself with the right kind of people, who actually had positive things to say to me, it was amazing how drastically my attitude toward both myself and life in general began to change. I began to believe in myself again, instead of suffocating my own abilities with fear and doubt. I began to live again.

Today, of course, I also have Todd. It was a cold winter day in December when we met; we had both shown up early to the Italian restaurant we were meeting at, and to this day, I've never known him to be early for anything other than that date and our wedding. He was wearing a Minnesota Twins shirt and stocking cap that day. Although I wasn't exactly a baseball fan, I was a fan of his sweet smile and his gentle manner. When we walked in the doors of the restaurant together, he took off his cap and flattened down his brown hair. Over the next couple of hours at dinner, I wondered why I had never liked brown eyes before. Our date ended at about 11:30 p.m., and only because we both had to work the next day. The next night we talked on the phone for over two hours. We've talked every day since.

If I would have met Todd a few years earlier, I would have understood what real love is like. Or, if I'd somehow been able to flash-forward and see a momentary glimpse of what our relationship would be like, I wouldn't have stayed in the horrible one I'd been in earlier.

But then again, maybe earlier just wasn't the right time for us. Todd has told me he thinks he remembers seeing me a year and a half before we actually met; he had been in a parade in the small town of Whoville that I mentioned earlier—a parade that I had also been at, watching. The parade was literally a week or two after I got out of that old horrible relationship, when I was still trying to put all of the little pieces of myself back together. He says he remembers seeing a girl sitting on the curb, wrapped up in a blanket. It was true that I had a blanket with me that day, and that I was sitting in the exact spot on the curb that he described for me. Some time after that, but still before we met, he remembers also seeing me in front of what he learned to be my parents' house, with my yellow car. He had been driving past the area to deliver a piece of farm equipment for his dad's dealership.

I guess neither of those times were the right times for us. On the day of the parade, he had still been in another relationship (with someone who clearly didn't have any of the amazing qualities of the person writing this book), and I was still just a bunch of broken pieces. I think we both had a lot of growing and learning to do before we could finally meet each other, so as not to taint the beautiful love we have today.

As I said in the last chapter, my husband is honest, even if he knows he's going to say something I might not like. He calls when he says he's going to call. If he says he's going to do something, I know that he will do it. He respects me wholly: He'll listen to what I have to say and try to understand where I'm coming from, even if he doesn't always agree. Physically, he knows that no matter how long we've been together, he doesn't own me or my body. Together, we're able to learn new things from each other, and encourage one another to continually grow, achieve our goals, and try to become better people.

Above all, I can honestly say that I trust him. I can be myself around him, and I know he understands who that person is. I feel even *more* like "me" when I'm with him, because when he looks at me, he doesn't see just a body, but a whole spectrum of wonderful attributes and abilities. He gets all my random jokes—even the ones that make some people think I'm just a little odd. When I'm with him, I feel good inside. I feel grounded. It feels right.

From the very beginning of our relationship, both of us have made it a point to set a solid foundation. If we get annoyed by something the other says or does, we talk about it and then try to see it from the other's point of view. If we start to feel a little hurt, we do our best to not take things personally, because we know neither of us would ever do anything to intentionally hurt the other. Again, we talk about it until we figure out what happened and how we can try to keep it from happening again in the future. Often we find that there has just been some kind of misunderstanding, so every time we talk, we learn a little bit more about each other. Just like in any relationship, things aren't perfect all the time—after all, we're only human! The important thing is knowing we can trust and depend on one another, and that we both genuinely love and respect each other. That's what matters.

So what's my point through all this relationship storytelling? The bottom line is this: The people you surround yourself with do have a *huge* impact on not only your recovery, but also your overall well-being. They can build you up, or break you down. This goes for relationships well beyond just the dating/married relationship, too—after all, some of the other people in your life can have just as big of an impact on you as a significant other.

Whether you're single, dating, or in a committed relationship, you have to know that the people you're spending your time with are enriching your life. You will only ever be as healthy as your relationships. This chapter will help you evaluate and build your bonds with others:

Evaluate Your Connections

Identify both the positive and negative influences in your life. Know how the people you spend your time with affect you. There are some people you have no choice but to be around, like those you work with or those who might cut in front of you in the line for your morning coffee. But when it comes to your friends, be aware of how they make you feel. You should usually feel better after being with them, not worse. If your friends are constantly saying mean or negative things, there are probably better people you could spend your time with.

During the darkest and loneliest part of my life, I didn't consider myself to be an attractive person because of some of the things my ex said to me. I dressed in drab colors and never bought anything nice for myself. I thought I was weak and dependent. Now, with Todd and with all of the other wonderful people I've added to my life, I feel good about myself both inside and out. My friends recognize the positive things I do and encourage me to keep working towards my goals, instead of criticizing me or reminding me of things that haven't gone my way.

Don't be afraid to approach people who might make good friends: Dr. Diana Repack, 46, from Pennsylvania, said she never would have hit it off with her husband if she hadn't become more assertive as a result of her recovery:

> *"My husband knows that I have a history of eating disorders and sometimes I talk about what I was like back then. One thing I am sure of is that if I had met my husband when my eating disorder was active, he never would have looked twice at me. I rarely smiled, and he is a friendly, outgoing person. I was the most negative person around, and he has a very optimistic view of life. Solid in my recovery at the time I met him, I was the one who struck up a conversation with him at a seminar at my university. I never would have approached him as the 'Eating disorder-me.' But he and the 'recovered me' make a great team, and we'll be celebrating 13 years of marriage this year."*

You never know what kind of amazing people you're going to meet once you recover!

Here are a few things to keep in mind when it comes to your friendships:

While it's important to make friends with people who can relate to your struggles, keep healthy boundaries. It's wonderful to connect with other people who are trying to recover from disordered eating and similar issues, because it helps to be able to talk to people who really understand what you're going through. However, you have to make sure those relationships aren't affecting you adversely. It will be hard for you to stick to your meal plan if the people you're talking to aren't staying on theirs. Just the same, if they have the tendency to talk about things like dieting or losing weight, it's going to be nearly impossible for you to not be thinking about it all the time, too. Make sure that you and anyone else you are talking to who is also in recovery, is just as committed to the process as you are.

Have a diverse group of friends. If you're like me and enjoy having a great deal of routine in your life, it's really refreshing to know someone a little more spontaneous, who can encourage you to shake things up a little from time to time. Friends with different hobbies can help you try new things. A good group of friends can really help you get your mind off of anything you might be dealing with throughout and even after your recovery.

Get connected and meet new people. If you'd like to create some healthy new relationships, try to get more actively involved in your community. It can be a little tough to start a friendship with that cheerful guy or girl who sits in front of you at church every now and then, but if you're consistently going to the same church volunteer group, it will be an entirely different story. It's a lot easier to get to know someone when you're seeing them on a regular basis, and once you know them better it will feel a little more natural to ask them to go do something with you. Here are a few places where you can get involved and meet people with common interests:

- Community service organizations
- Volunteer work with an agency you respect
- Church groups
- Community sports leagues
- Classes at your gym
- Classes at a local college
- Play groups (for those who are parents)
- Political organizations
- Your city's Chamber of Commerce
- Local writers' groups, or other special interest groups
- Part-time jobs (working somewhere fun!)

Check out your local newspaper's website for listings of community events and club meetings to get a better idea of what's being offered in your community. If you're ambitious, you could also consider starting a local group for something you enjoy, like crafting, cooking, hiking, or going to sporting events. This obviously takes quite a bit more work than simply joining a club that already exists, but all of the things you'll be doing to get the group started will be additional opportunities for you to get out and meet new people. See Chapter Three for more tips on starting a special interest group.

In each of your relationships, be honest with yourself about how you and the other person make each other feel, by asking yourself these questions:

- Does one of you tell the other how they should spend their time?
- Does one of you try to "punish" the other for saying something they don't like?
- Does one of you use threats to get the other to behave a certain way?
- Does one tell the other who they specifically may or may not spend time with?
- Do you call each other names, put each other down, or otherwise make each other feel bad about yourselves?
- Do you raise your voice or use physical force when you're upset with one another?
- Does one of you try to get the other to do things that are not in their best interest?
- Do one or both of you ever feel nervous or afraid around the other?
- Is one of you afraid to talk to the other sometimes, for fear of how they might react?

If you answered "yes" to one or more of these questions, it's a definite sign that this relationship may not be a positive one for you or the other person. Relationships that involve abusive elements such as fear, control, or isolation will negatively influence you in other areas of your life. Your recovery, overall health, and satisfaction in life will be compromised if you continue to stay in a relationship with these kinds of dynamics. As I said earlier, I had to get out of the relationship I was in because it was crushing me emotionally. It wasn't until I began making more positive connections that I had the support I needed to finally recover from my eating disorder and begin experiencing a more fulfilling life. However, because I can't give any specific advice on how to deal with *your* individual situation, I highly suggest you talk to a counselor or therapist about your circumstances. He or she will be able to help you take an honest assessment of your relationship and begin figuring out what you can do that will benefit you the most.

What if you answered "No" to all those questions? Even if your relationship is healthy, is it as supportive as it could be?

Ask yourself these questions about you and your friend/partner/family member:

- Do you and the other person support one another emotionally?
- Do you make each other feel good about yourselves?
- Do you find yourself often laughing with each other?
- Are you able to communicate with one another without fear?

- Do you accept each other's feelings as valid, rather than telling each other you're somehow "wrong" for feeling them?
- Are you able to talk about both silly and serious things?
- Are you respectful of each other, even when you disagree on something?
- Do you listen to one another?
- Are you able to compromise, without one person feeling like they're always giving in?
- Do you challenge each other to grow and achieve your goals?
- In general, are you happy together?
- Are you truly able to be yourself around this person?
- Do you trust this person?

If you answered "yes" to all of these questions, it is likely that this is a very healthy relationship. This is the kind of relationship that will support you through both recovery and any other bumps in life. So what if you answered "no" to some of the questions? Any negative answers may signal an area where your relationship could use a little work. Take a look at what some of those areas may be and consider talking to your friend/partner/family member about how you can improve them. In any relationship, communication and the willingness to work together are keys.

Make your "Love (or Friendship) List." Looking for a simple and effective way to screen potential dates? Or, if you're not interested or ready for the dating scene or are already in a committed relationship, do you need a way to evaluate potential friends? This list will help you:

Get out a sheet of paper and make four columns. In the first column, list all of the qualities or values you absolutely want in a relationship, like someone of the same religion or political view, someone with good family values, or someone who goes to church regularly—anything that is really important to you.

In the second column list all of the qualities you'd like to have, such as someone who likes dogs, someone who works out regularly, or someone who enjoys staying up late on the weekends.

In the third column list all of the things you would prefer your potential date or friend to *not* have or be, such as someone who loves horror movies if you're more into comedies, or someone who hates fish if you're a sushi fanatic.

In the fourth column write anything you absolutely do *not* want, like someone who smokes or who never cleans his or her house (What you put in these columns is obviously going to be different depending on whether you're evaluating someone you'd like to date or simply be friends with—after all, it's a little bit different to be friends with someone who's a sloppy housekeeper than it is to eventually wind up sharing a home with them!).

Love/Friendship List Example

Must Have	Would Like	Would Not Like	Absolutely Do Not Want
Someone who…	**Someone who...**	**Someone who…**	**Someone who…**
Loves family	Enjoys riding bike	Always texts instead of calling	Lies to me
Loves kids	Likes seafood	Swears a lot	Puts me down
Supports my religious beliefs	Makes me laugh	Is lazy	Doesn't get along with my family
Is open and easy to talk to	Likes to read	Is messy	Is rude
Listens to me	Likes to cook	Is usually late	Is hard to talk to
Respects me	Volunteers in the community	Gets annoyed by some of my friends	Doesn't get my sense of humor
Is honest	Enjoys gardening		Doesn't like to try new things
Likes animals	Likes going for walks		Doesn't like to travel
Is outgoing	Has a good imagination		
Is polite	Has a good job		
Is hard-working			

When you've filled out all of the columns, do an honest comparison between your date and everything you've written down. That hottie you met last week might not seem so attractive a year down the road when he still won't let your dog touch him. I'm not saying opposites can't attract, but from my own experience it wasn't until after I found someone highly compatible with me that my love life became what I'd always dreamed of it becoming. That being said, everyone is different; it's up to you to decide what you will and won't accept in a relationship. Use your "Love (or Friendship) List" as your guide.

Once you've figured out who your top supportive people are, check out these tips for nurturing your relationships with them:

Keep Your Relationships Happy

Be open about your eating disorder with the people who matter. Even though it can be really hard, talking to the people you love about what you're dealing with will help them understand you more. The more they understand you, the better your relationship will become, and the more they'll be able to support you when you're having a rough time. I opened up to my husband about my eating disorder shortly after we began dating. I don't remember exactly how the conversation came up the first time, but I do remember feeling a little bit "on edge" about the whole thing. It wasn't easy to talk to him at first, because like so many other people, he had all kinds of preconceived notions about what it meant to have an eating disorder. He thought many of the same things that your loved ones might think, like eating disorders only being about superficial things like food or wanting to be the skinniest person in the room. Our first few conversations definitely weren't easy. He was always respectful and tried to be as supportive as possible, but I could tell that he just didn't "get it."

It wasn't until he came to watch one of my eating disorder presentations (based on an early draft of this book) at a local university that things finally sort of "clicked" for him. In the coming weeks and months I was able to explain to him many of the complexities that went along with some of my struggles. It took a good deal of talking, listening, and patience on both of our parts, but it was well worth it in the end. We found that even though he has never had an eating disorder, there are many thoughts and feelings we do have that are very similar. It's because we've *both* made an effort to understand each other better that we're now able to talk openly and freely with one another about *anything*, and know that we'll always be supported. This openness has created an amazing amount of trust between us, and has turned my husband into the closest and truest friend I ever could have imagined for myself.

Be open to new ideas from others. Julia, 23, from Worcestershire,

England, said her life opened up once she learned to be more open to other people's perspectives:

> *"My eating disorder sub-consciously convinced me that I didn't need other people and that MY perspective (albeit anorexic) was the only way to see myself and the rest of the world. Actually, learning to open up and trust in other people's viewpoints of life, and particularly their far more realistic perspective of myself, has led to so many possibilities that I previously would not have even dreamed could have existed."*

Be yourself. I know—how cliché does that sound, right? But it's true. Angela, 29, from California said it's now a goal of hers to be completely genuine with both herself and others, and that her relationships are now based more on honesty than they were in the past:

> *"I've found that the more genuine I am with myself, the more people like me for ME, and the less I feel like I have to be someone I'm not, or remake myself into someone different so I'm accepted. When I was able to accept myself it was absolutely freeing."*

Jan Lockert, 53, from Ohio, said her ability to be open and accepting of herself gave a new depth to her relationships:

> *"Before recovery, my relationships were guarded, very superficial, and uncomfortable. I was terrified of what others were thinking about me…I wore a 'mask' of joy and complete satisfaction, and I was forever trying to make others happy at any cost to myself…I felt obligated to never allow others to see my 'imperfections,' yet my emaciated appearance told it all. I now love meeting new people and developing open and emotionally honest relationships. I learned during recovery, with frequent reminders from my therapist, that by taking the risk to reveal myself, I was also giving the other person the freedom to be open."*

Be assertive and share your feelings. I'm not talking about telling the person next to you on the subway about your menstrual cramps, but if there's something that's really bothering you, make sure you talk about it so it doesn't grow into something huge that might come between you. Also tell people if there are certain things they talk about, like dieting or weight loss, that trigger unhealthy thoughts for you. Your conversations with them should be a positive experience, and not a source of discomfort.

Remember to say "Thank you" to your loved ones, even for the little things that don't seem to "matter." When I first started dating my husband, I was amazed by how polite he was: He thanked me for our phone calls, and for spending time with him. He thanked me for things like picking up a piece of litter on the sidewalk or holding a door open for someone in front of us. By doing that, he told me that not only did he appreciate the things I was doing, but he appreciated *me*. His kindness really made an impact on me, and so ever since then I've tried to do the same for him. I thank him for the hug he gives me when he comes home from school, and for calling me during the day to let me know what's going on with his busy schedule later. My husband has told me one of the things he loves about me is that I'm so polite, but the secret is that even though I've always said "please" and "thank you," he's the one who really drove home the importance of those words for me. It makes a big difference in our relationship to know that we are always appreciated for all of the little things we do for each other. And it also has its other benefits: Thanking someone for doing something we like is the best way to make sure they keep doing it in the future!

Turn your disagreements into *discussions* instead of fights. When my husband and I don't see eye to eye on something, we turn our conversation about it into a discussion rather than an argument. We both make an honest effort to listen and try to understand each other's perspectives, instead of raising our voices and simply trying to prove the other wrong. Often we'll find that even if we disagree on something, we're able to learn more about both the topic and each other, and find some common ground. **Respect for the other person and their viewpoint is essential in any discussion.** As long as that respect is mutual, discussions are much more likely to be productive and end well. **Timing is also important:** Don't try to start a serious discussion when someone is in the middle of a big project, on their way out the door, or already upset about something else. They also might not be able to talk about some things until they've had a chance to think and figure out how they feel on their own first.

Don't be afraid to say "I'm sorry" or "I was wrong." Even though it can be really hard at first, it gets easier. Saying those phrases helps you and your loved ones feel more like a "team"—not people who always have to be on two different sides of the battlefield.

If you and your family are having trouble talking, **consider going to family therapy.** A counselor or therapist will be able to help you and your family members learn to talk about tough issues in a productive way, or simply learn to communicate with one another better. Rachelle, 23, from Arizona said that even though her family is very supportive, there were some issues related to her disorder that weren't resolved until they worked on them together in therapy. She said they now have better relationships because they've reached a place where they're better able to understand one another.

Make healthy goals with the people you love. You're not the only one who's trying to make positive changes, so don't feel like the focus needs to be solely on you. Maybe you and your mom both want to start following a meal plan, or maybe you and your sister can start going to the gym together to make sure you get in a good workout without overdoing it. Be a cheerleader for your boyfriend who's trying to quit smoking, while he encourages you to make healthier food choices.

Make weekly "dates." It's important to stay connected throughout (and after!) your recovery, so you don't start to slip back into old thoughts and behaviors. Make it a point to schedule regular times during the week when you can visit with the people in your support system about how you're doing, rather than waiting until things come up at times when you're unprepared to talk, or in the wrong mood to talk about them.

Figure out who you're going to talk to every week, and when: Meet a friend for coffee every Tuesday afternoon, and let your mom know you'll be coming over on Sunday mornings. You'll be more likely to make the right decisions just knowing that these meetings are coming up, and the lines of communication (about what might be triggering you, what fears you may be having, accomplishments, etc.) will always be open for you!

Remember that **your loved ones aren't responsible for your emotions or your recovery.** They're wonderful to have as support, but ultimately it's up to you how you feel. A few years ago, I was lying on my parents' living room floor and trembling. I had begun to panic after thinking about moving out of their house and living alone. I was afraid of the idea of not having my parents with me in case something bad ever happened to me. My poor mom looked down at me and then said softly, "You know I can't do anything for you right now, right? I'm not *doing* anything for you."

My mom wasn't saying this to be mean; she was trying to get the point across that I was the only one who could learn to control my panic attacks and my other emotions. My mom's words have stayed with me since that day. Now whenever I start to feel nervous or sad, I'm able to upcycle my thoughts so they don't just keep spiraling downward like a giant snowball.

If you're struggling with your emotions, remember to lean on your counselor, because he or she is trained to help you. It's important to talk to your family and friends about how you're feeling, but try to make sure you're not always dwelling on the negative when you're with them!

Your relationships will naturally improve as you progress through recovery. Amy Pettengill, 27, from New Hampshire said it's thanks to her recovery that she began being able to have real relationships again:

> *"I have had the honor of being a real friend, sister, daughter, aunt, cousin, niece, etc. When I was active in my eating disorder I was unable to hold an active role in any relationship, because I was too focused on my obsessions and intense fears. If you were having a conversation with me when I was active in my eating disorder, I'm sorry, but I wasn't paying attention—most of the time I was focused on my eating disorder, food, fat, etc. That is not the case now. I am able to participate in*

conversations and be emotionally available for my friends and family. I can go out to eat and not have a panic attack. I want to hang out with people today, instead of staying isolated."

Relationships are an entirely different thing after recovery. They're brighter, richer, and deeper. They're more fun and more fulfilling. For me, they bring a genuine kind of happiness that can comfort me no matter what I'm dealing with.

Remember that other people's negative moods often have nothing to do with you. Everyone is human, which means there are going to be times when the people you care about just aren't quite feeling—or acting—their best. My husband and I have always been very sensitive to one another's subtlest behaviors. Even early on in our dating relationship, we could always tell when the other person was feeling a little "off." If I was quiet because I hadn't gotten enough sleep the night before, he would wonder if I was upset with him. If he had had a bad day at work and seemed a little distressed, I started to worry that I had said or done something that irritated him. We would then play off of each other's negative moods until something really *was* wrong between us!

My hubby and I have learned to ask each other what's going on, rather than just immediately taking each other's moods personally and then starting to feel pretty annoyed or upset ourselves. Sometimes we need to just give each other a little bit of time and space to think about what's really bothering us, before we try to talk about it.

Know that relationships change over time. Relationships change because life is always changing. You may need more support from someone early on in your recovery, while they may need a little extra love after a job loss or if they're diagnosed with a health issue of their own. What's important is that you **keep the lines of communication open about what each of you can do to support each other and keep your relationship strong.** Every once in awhile, set aside some time to ask your loved ones these questions:

1. How are you feeling about our relationship?

2. What do you like? What don't you like?

3. What could we improve, and how?

4. Is there anything else you'd like to talk about?

It does take some effort to actually ask these questions, but it's really minimal when you consider the benefits you gain from it. As long as you and your loved ones are both willing to talk openly, you'll keep your relationship at its best.

Your ability to love yourself greatly impacts your ability to love others. Arielle Lee Bair, 27, from Pennsylvania said it was only because she learned to love herself that she was able to love her husband when he entered into her life:

> *"I was able to share my past and my life—details and issues, too—and feel comfortable and unashamed. I was able to give my all in a relationship, because I wasn't preoccupied with food, weight, or numbers. I was able to be real in my relationship, because I had come to terms with what was inside of me. I was able to accept love and carry it with me, instead of feeling that I did not fully deserve it. I was able to stand in front of a dressing room mirror in my wedding gown and smile, because I looked healthy and happy. And I was able to walk down the aisle on my wedding day knowing that I was giving myself a shot at something completely worthwhile and loving every minute of it, because there was only room in me for happiness, not self-hate or obsession or fear."*

Fill yourself with positive, upcycled feelings about yourself, so there isn't room for any of that old junk that just keeps you stuck and miserable. The choice is yours.

Last, remember that **although your relationships can have a huge impact on your life, they will never define who YOU are.** It will always be up to you to choose your attitude, make positive choices, and treat other people well. Also, if you're not in a romantic relationship right now, **make it a point to never refer to yourself as single: Do as I did and call yourself "independent" instead!** After all, it's better to be independent than to be with someone who doesn't make you feel good, respect you, or treat you the way you deserve to be treated. You are just as important and special as anyone else, and you can definitely be just as happy!

The next topic is one that's nearly impossible to avoid. Unless you've never talked to a single person about eating disorders in your entire life, you know that there are all kinds of misconceptions about them, *and* about the people who experience them. You're more than likely going to run into at least one person who says something ignorant to you about either someone else's or your eating disorder. Here's how to respond:

What to Do When Someone Says Something Dumb

First things first: As tough as it is, **try not to take it personally. Usually people just don't know better.** Before I had an eating disorder myself, I was one of those people who used to laugh at jokes I heard about people with eating disorders. I didn't know what eating disorders or those who suffer from them are really like. Like so many others, I thought people who had them were just extremely shallow and vain. I had no clue how complex they actually are, and how truly sweet and loving so many of those who suffer from them are.

Ashley Devitt, 18, from Florida said that people often won't realize how unhelpful some of their comments are until you talk to them:

> *"People will say unhelpful comments such as, 'Wow you've gained weight; good job!' but you just have to understand that they think they are being supportive…family and friends aren't always perfect. They will make mistakes, trigger you, and perhaps feed the eating disorder even more. Instead of getting mad, it is essential that you tell them what they can do to improve: After all, how can they change if they don't know what they're doing to upset you in the first place?"*

Be proactive: **Make a list of "DO NOT SAY" phrases and give it to family members,** along with recommending books, like Ashley did. Here are some examples of potentially triggering comments to include on your list (yours may be similar or completely different):

- "You have such a healthy appetite now!"
- "You've gained weight."
- "You don't look like a twig (or a skeleton, or skinny, etc.) anymore."
- "You are curvy."
- "You don't exercise as much as you used to."

After you give the list to your loved ones, explain that the statements on them make you feel uncomfortable. Let them know how they can rephrase their words into statements that are a little better thought out, such as "You look full of energy!" instead of "You look so much better now that you've gained weight!", or "I love being able to enjoy a relaxing meal with you now," instead of "I love how much more you eat now!"

Don't thank anyone for compliments about weight gain (or anything else) that you don't truly appreciate. Ashley said that after recovering, some of her relatives made a lot of comments about the weight she had gained. Instead of thanking them, she simply would nod her head and say something like, "Yes, I've been working on that," or "Yes, I have." She said she never felt obligated to say anything more than that if she didn't want to.

Give healthy answers to negative questions. Ashley said that even today when she gets a question about her weight, she replies by saying, "'I try not to focus on numbers, because they really don't matter in the long run. As long as I'm eating healthily, I should be in a healthy weight range." She also doesn't answer if she's asked about her lowest weight. Take a cue from Ashley and **don't talk about numbers, even if people ask**

specifically for them. It's not healthy for people to be making comparisons or getting unhealthy ideas about weights, calorie consumption, fat grams, exercise minutes, etc.—especially when an eating disorder has been involved.

If someone says something that really bothers you and you're not sure how to respond right away, **take a time out.** Go somewhere quiet for awhile, take a brisk walk, or call a friend to vent. If someone asks you something personal about your struggles or about something sensitive that you don't feel comfortable answering, **respect your own privacy.** I think it is important to share information if you think it might help someone, but you don't owe random people any explanations beyond that.

If someone says something that embarrasses or upsets you, remember that **things can only get awkward if you allow them to.** If someone says something rude or ignorant to you, whether they mean anything by it or not, you have the choice to not let it affect you. Go ahead and scream into your pillow later, but try to brush it off in the moment if you can. It will be a whole lot easier to deal with in the long run.

Use rude and ignorant comments as an opportunity to be an advocate. The only way people will change their mindsets is if you educate them. Correct them if they're repeating misconceptions about eating disorders or the people who have them.

At the end of the day, remember that **there are a lot of people who can relate to what you're going through.** Even if they've never had a clear-cut eating disorder, there are plenty of people who struggle with their own eating and body image disturbances, or other addictions. They may not exactly understand everything you're dealing with, but they probably can relate on some level.

Once I stopped isolating myself and worrying about all of the "flaws" I imagined others were seeing in me, I had a wonderful revelation: I realized that amazingly enough, people really do like me as a person. They laugh at my ridiculous jokes. They smile when I walk into a room. They feel better after talking to me.

There's no way I would ever go back to the way my life was before. I can't tell you how amazingly my relationships have improved since I finally really opened up to those I love: I have never felt closer to my dad—I never would have imagined how similarly we think, or how much I appreciate being able to talk to him about so many things now. I can talk to my sister, brother, and mom like I never could before. I know I can count on anyone in my family being there if I need them for something. I also trust my husband in a way I never thought possible. With him, I've discovered a kind of love and kinship that I never would have thought possible before.

I feel so blessed knowing there are people with whom I can be completely honest, without being rejected and without them thinking any less of me. It was throughout all of those really rough spots that I was able to realize how much they actually *love* me, unconditionally—and it's with this understanding that I've been able to heal as fully as I have over the years.

Take a leap of faith, and open up. Find the people in your life who truly do love you and who will be there for you when it counts (or even just be with you to watch a lame movie on a Sunday afternoon). You don't ever have to feel alone again!

Here are this chapter's journal questions, followed by the family and Q & A segments:

Journal Questions

1. What kinds of relationships would I like to form?
2. What would I like to receive from these relationships?
3. What kinds of good qualities can I contribute to a relationship?

Tips for Friends & Family

Plan a fun outing with your loved one.

Plan to do something fun with your loved one, that doesn't have anything to do with their eating disorder: Go on a movie date, take a walk in the park, or plan a game night. Go camping, have a bonfire, and tell ghost stories. Spend some time reconnecting, and remind your loved one what life is really about—living, loving, laughing, and experiencing!

Practice good communication.

All those effective communication skills you've heard about will come in especially handy now: As Cheryl Kerrigan, 41, from Massachusetts said, it's important to use "I" statements rather than "you" statements when talking about sensitive subjects, "so as not to come across as attacking or threatening." Also remember to speak calmly, and if possible, talk to your loved one about those tough subjects at times when he or she is more likely to be relaxed.

Make it a point to talk to your loved one every day—both about their recovery and their day in general. Open and honest communication is the key to good relationships, and it's through good relationships that people are able to heal. Kristen, 25, from Wisconsin said that as long as you keep the lines of communication open, your loved one will know they can always come to you to talk if they're struggling with something. She said, "I am a firm believer in the saying that we are 'only as sick as our secrets.' If the sufferer can open up about their 'secrets,' it is a huge burden off of their shoulders, and it is one less thing working against them."

Be unconditional.

The best thing you can do for your loved one will always be to simply be there for them and let them know you believe in them. Kelly, 28, from New Jersey, shared how her boyfriend's support impacted her recovery:

> *"When I began dating my boyfriend, I told him (on the second date) that I had struggled with an eating disorder. I wanted to be upfront with him from the start. At that time, though, he couldn't really grasp how serious it was. Within a year, I had a major relapse, and I brought him down with me. There were many arguments over food, and the love and joy that we had in our relationship was overcome with anxiety over meals. The tension grew between us.*
>
> *"This relapse was different, though: I wanted recovery. Although the recovery process was slow, I continued to fight for it. I invited my boyfriend with me to my therapy sessions, and he took an active role in my recovery, while still acknowledging that I was the only one who could (and needed) to do the work. One night, which is forever burned in my mind, he sat with me in the car and asked me what was going on with work. That conversation still brings tears to my eyes: He knew that it wasn't about food. He knew that something was bothering me so deeply, and that I just didn't know how to express it. He could see that I was in pain, and he reached out his hand to me to walk with me through the troubled times.*
>
> *"Slowly, I made progress. My boyfriend was there with me, every step of the way. He encouraged me with things like, 'Hey, I've noticed that you are smiling a lot more. That's good to see.' He also encouraged me by reminding me that recovery is a process. He didn't expect perfection; he just wanted to see that I was trying. I reassured him that sometimes I just need a hug or a listening ear. I confided in him when I was trying a 'risky' food, and he was right there to offer a smile or a gentle hand squeeze under the table.*
>
> *"Today is much different. A few months ago, I decided to ask him how he felt about my recovery. I knew how I felt—I felt as though anorexia was nearly a distant memory. His response took my breath away: 'I don't even realize that you have an eating disorder, anymore. I am proud of how hard you worked in recovery. I know you might still have the thoughts, but you don't let them hold you back, and that shows what a strong person you are. You are so much happier and energetic and fun.'*

"Hearing those words, that he was proud of me—Me?! Wow, for the first time since this dreadful disorder entered my life, I felt like I could (and was well on my way to) conquer my eating disorder."

Questions Friends & Family Should Ask

1. What are some helpful things for you to hear from me? What's not helpful?

2. What can you and I do tonight (or tomorrow, this weekend, etc.) for fun?

3. What do you like best about our relationship? What would you like to improve, and how do you think we could improve it?

Journal Questions for Friends & Family

1. How is my relationship with my loved one improving? What are some things we can do to make it even better?

2. How are we at communicating? What could be improved?

3. How can I show my love? What do I need in return? (Tip: I highly recommend reading *The Five Love Languages* by Gary Chapman if you haven't already. This will give you some great insight as to how to respond to this question!)

Q & A with Carolyn Costin, MFT, M.ED., and Keesha Broome, M.A., MFT

Q: How do I know if I'm ready to get involved in a romantic relationship?

A: There is no magic formula for knowing if or when you are ready for a relationship. Your recovery should be your first priority and romantic relationships naturally challenge this hierarchy. Relationships are also often the place where all of our "stuff" comes up. Your relationship with yourself is the basis for your recovery. So you need to be able to give yourself the space and energy to foster this.

Until you have a firm grasp on healthy thought patterns and behaviors, it is important to have undivided time to focus on your own healing. However, relationships sometimes just happen, and we do not feel in control to let this person pass by. Be honest! You have already spent way too much time hiding your feelings and your disorder from others. You definitely need people around you who can support you, and this is not possible if you cannot tell them the truth. If you cannot tell them the truth, this is a good sign that you are not ready to be in a relationship.

6 Make Your Order: Finding harmony with your meal plan

"A bad habit never disappears miraculously; it's an undo-it-yourself project."

– *Abigail Van Buren*

When I was 10 years old and running through the sprinklers, I didn't think very much about what I was going to eat. If I wanted a milkshake, I had one. If I wanted mayonnaise on my sandwich, I smeared it on. I helped myself to Grandma's brownies without beating myself up about it later. I ate broccoli and brussels sprouts because I liked *them*, and not just their calorie counts.

It wasn't until my freshman year in high school that I began to think about what I was eating a little bit more—that is to say, I stopped letting myself just eat what I wanted to eat, when I wanted to eat it. I thought my natural weight was just too heavy, and I wanted to change it. I started to say no to my grandma's special chocolate chip cookies and only took tiny slices of the yummy lasagna I made for my family at dinner. I started eating skimpy breakfasts and stopped eating snacks after school (I feel sad and hungry just writing this now!).

A couple of years later I started working out. I began to notice that I could eat more when I worked out, and still maintain my weight. I started working out more. I started eating a lot more. I began eating all of the things I used to love, but that I had deprived myself of for so long—except that now I was eating about twice as much of it as I used to. I definitely wasn't paying attention to my body's hunger signals!

It was only a matter of time before I noticed that I had "suddenly" put back on all of the weight I had lost, and then some. I was 17 at the time. I remember putting on a pair of my jeans and realizing that they were much tighter than before. I panicked—how had that happened? I was frustrated with both myself and the fact that I didn't think *I* could eat like "normal people" without getting "fat." I thought *other* people could eat things like brownies and cake and pizza without gaining weight, but that I clearly couldn't. It didn't seem fair. I didn't *want* to always have to just watch other people eating fun foods, without being able to enjoy the experience right along with them. I didn't want to spend the rest of my life on a restrictive diet, but I didn't want to spend it being overweight, either.

That was when I began my struggle with bulimia. I thought I finally had figured out the "perfect" answer to my food and body problems. I thought I could eat whatever I wanted, without having to worry about my weight. What I *hadn't* realized was how much bingeing and purging for over three years would actually mess up both my mind and body: My anxiety and depression skyrocketed, and I could never concentrate on anything for very long before I started to think about food. I was constantly exhausted, and my muscles always felt weak and tingly.

When I finally began attempting to recover from bulimia, I questioned every single thing I put into my mouth. I was afraid I'd lose control over my eating if I just let myself have what I wanted. I had also read so many random diet articles that I was afraid if I ever ate anything not on my "approved" list of foods, I might suddenly morph into some freakish, cellulite-encrusted version of myself.

Rather than going to a dietitian and trying to learn how to follow a balanced eating plan, I began obsessively planning and recording every little thing I ate. By the time I was 25, I was eating the same boring things every day, at exactly the same times and in exactly the same order. Lunch was always precisely at 1:10 p.m.—not 1:00 or even 1:09 (1:11 maybe would have been okay, but only because I thought it meant I was exercising self-control). I didn't like eating out, or even eating with other people at all, because that would have completely thrown off my eating routine. I cherished my routine, because it felt comfortable and safe; I thought it was the only thing that would keep me from overeating.

Before I knew what was happening, my recovery from bulimia had gradually turned into a battle with anorexia. Needless to say, I had a lot to learn about both normal eating and how my body worked before I could ever really recover. **You know what helped me finally stop obsessing about food, and start living my life?** As annoying as it might be to hear, **I had to just eat.** I had to eat food I didn't want to eat, and often I had to eat more of it than I wanted. In time my hunger signals normalized, I stopped worrying so much about everything I was eating, and I found myself actually enjoying my life instead of spending every minute thinking about what I was (or wasn't) going to eat next.

In time, **I learned that all of my old fears about eating were wrong:** When I was 17, I hadn't gained weight because I was eating "bad" foods, but because I hadn't been paying attention to my body's hunger signals while I was eating them. I was probably eating five brownies, instead of the one or two that would have satisfied me. I didn't understand the balance that comes with normal eating, and I definitely didn't trust my body to help me figure it out, either. It wasn't until several years later that I finally began letting myself just *eat*, without overthinking everything or worrying about what was going to "happen" to my body. **I had to learn to become an ally with my body, instead of trying unsuccessfully to control it.**

When you're trying to get on a meal plan again, even if you feel like you're starving and want to binge and eat forever, rest assured that those feelings *won't* last forever. **As long as you're making an honest effort to listen to your body, you will learn to recognize and respond to its signals.** You will also feel less ravenous once your body starts getting the nourishment that it requires. It takes a little bit of time, but once you start to figure out that balance, you'll feel better than ever. For me, eating almost feels as natural as it did when I was younger. The only difference is that now I'm more educated about nutrition and food choices, so I eat based both on my tastes and what's best for me. I try to eat healthy because it's good for my body, but I sure as heck include room for some fun foods, too!

So what does a healthy diet look like?

How to Eat

First things first: **There really is no such thing as a "normal" diet**. It seems like every time you pick up a magazine or peruse the internet, you see something about certain foods you absolutely should or should not include in your diet. The truth is, there are lots of healthy people who probably eat completely different things, depending on where they live and what tastes good to them. The key lies in eating a balance of different foods so your body gets all of the nutrients it needs. I don't really like milk except in my cereal, but I do eat a lot of yogurt and cheese to make sure I get enough calcium. I also make sure I get a balance of protein, fats, and carbohydrates at every meal. As long as you're staying relatively mindful—not obsessive!—about what you're eating, and trying to keep a good variety of foods in your meal plan, your diet is more than likely going to be pretty well-rounded.

Thecla, 24, from Illinois, had a great description of what a normal, healthy diet is:

> *"...being able to eat what you want, when you want, and not feeling guilty about it or thinking that you have to make up for it. It's being able to eat a variety of foods without restricting certain foods just because you fear them. It's taking control instead of giving the control to the food. It's being able to eat the piece of birthday cake with your friends, and then still eating dinner later without obsessing over what it's going to 'do' to you. It's being able to splurge every now and then without thinking about the calories, because it all evens out in the end. It's listening to your body to know when you are full, when you are craving something, and when*

you need more. A normal, healthy diet is being able to sit down to a meal with your family or friends and laughing and having a good time, and at the end of the meal having no idea what everyone else ate and not really thinking about what you just ate either, because it's just food and you were having a good time."

A normal diet includes eating a little bit differently from day to day, depending on how you're feeling and what you're doing. **You may be pretty uncomfortable with the idea of normal eating at first**, especially if you're used to restricting your food, or purging after eating what would be considered an ordinary amount by others. That's why I think it's important that you **don't confuse normal eating with bingeing:** A binge is different from normal eating because it involves eating a larger amount of food in a small amount of time than might typically be expected of others in similar circumstances. Having an extra brownie or two at a work potluck is not a binge, and neither is enjoying some popcorn at the movie theater every once in awhile when you're not really hungry. If you begin to feel triggered after having an extra treat or two, reframe your thoughts and remind yourself that you are eating normally—*not* bingeing. Once you begin allowing yourself to have that extra brownie (or whatever other foods you may not have allowed yourself to have in the past) from time to time, you will start to notice yourself beginning to feel more and more in control of your eating decisions.

Going along with that, remember that even though we use the word "diet" sometimes, **your diet is not actually "a diet," because healthy eating doesn't have any "rules."** There are some choices that are nutritionally better than others, but unless you have a real allergy or other reason to avoid certain foods, nothing is off limits. As long as you're listening to your physical and emotional hunger cues, your body will find its ideal weight (See Chapter Eight for more on finding—and feeling comfortable with!—your healthy weight).

If you haven't already done so, **visit a dietitian to make a meal plan to fit *your* lifestyle.** None of the magazines or internet articles will be able to tell you what's right specifically for you, and many of them actually have a lot of misinformation about certain foods. I spent years avoiding pasta like it was poisonous, before I realized that it actually can be part of a really healthy diet. Your dietitian can help you create a plan that includes food you actually like and that will help you meet your nutritional needs. Having a meal plan will keep you on track with your goals and help you avoid over-thinking every single thing you eat, so you can focus on more important things!

Use resources such as http://www.choosemyplate.gov/ to educate yourself about healthy eating. This website is from the United States Department of Agriculture, and I love it because it has all kinds of helpful information about what a balanced diet consists of, as well as healthy eating tips, examples of serving sizes, and even individualized daily food plans. This is a place where you can go for accurate nutrition information and learn about the health benefits of eating foods from *every* food group, without any gimmicks or fad diets. Use this resource, but also remember that it is *not* a substitute for a real person who is knowledgeable about your individual nutritional needs!

Include all kinds of foods in your meal plan. Don't just stick to the same foods you've been eating over and over again. **Be honest with yourself about any dietary restrictions you may have for yourself, whether it be not eating meat, sugar, dairy, gluten, etc.** What are your reasons for not eating those foods? Do you have a true health or moral reason for not eating them, or are you cutting them out of your diet as a way to control your weight? Do you have a true allergy or intolerance to them, or are you simply afraid to eat them? Check out the next chapter (Chapter Seven) for some tips on defeating your food fears and getting a healthy variety back in your diet.

Pick a weekly food-related "intervention." Just like the interventions mentioned in Chapter One, these are challenges that you can gradually incorporate into your diet, with the help of the people who are supporting you. Each week, choose one of the interventions from the list below (or make up one of your own). This list was given to me by Registered Dietitian Barbara Truitt:

- Find a slogan, phrase, or affirmation to use before a meal or challenging event that involves food. One client used to say, "Just do it."
- Recite a prayer, either out loud or to yourself.
- Tell the person you are eating with to keep you engaged in conversation.
- If you eat your meals alone, go to a nice surrounding (i.e. patio, balcony, park, the pool) and focus on the birds, clouds, planes.
- Plan your meals in a menu-style and review them with your nutritionist.
- Fully understand the food groups; it is important to know that one slice of bread is equal to 1/3 cup of rice or 1/2 cup cereal, 1/2 cup cooked pasta, etc.
- Remind yourself that your meal plan is safe.
- When struggling, tell your nutritionist and/or therapist that you need to do a couple of MSTs (Mealtime Support Therapies—where you eat a meal from your meal plan with the nutritionist or therapist. See Barbara's Q & A section towards the end of this chapter for more information).
- Practice deep breathing before the meal.

- Put your utensils down every two or three bites.
- Drink liquids after the meal, rather than before or during.
- During a meal, when you find yourself getting anxious, take a deep breath, and begin eating in a normal pattern (i.e. one bite of chicken, then one bite of green beans, one bite of rice, go back to the chicken, etc.).
- Avoid consuming all of one particular food group one at a time.
- Play soft, non-lyrical music in the background.
- Turn your phone on silent and do not answer the phone during a meal—you may be tempted to use this as an excuse to not finish the meal.
- Avoid eating a meal with those who cause tension or badger you to eat, or talk about how little you eat.
- Though it sounds silly, be sure you are wearing comfortable clothes.
- After your meal, say your prayer and take a 10-minute vitality walk (this will help the feeling of fullness pass more easily).
- Ask your nutritionist to do a home session with you and show you simple, basic cooking skills.
- Ask your nutritionist to help you grocery shop once in awhile.
- Refresh your ability to read food labels with your nutritionist.
- When eating challenging foods, refrain from "dissecting" them.
- Remember to eat sandwiches and wraps with your hands.
- Get into the habit of eating salads as a salad, rather than picking them apart and "dipping" each vegetable into a serving of salad dressing.

Let your family know about your meal plan. Kelly, 28, from New Jersey, pointed out the fact that recovery is an adjustment for family members just as much as it is for those in recovery; she showed her family her meal plans and made a grocery list before she left treatment. She added that the more open you are with your loved ones, the more comfortable they'll feel talking about it, and the whole process overall, with you.

It will take time and a conscious effort to change some of your habits, like picking certain ingredients out of your pasta or throwing away pieces of your sandwiches before you've finished eating them. **Stay consistent.** Every single day is important to you in the long-term. As long as you're following your plan, you'll be able to stay on track without over-thinking everything you eat.

Make a schedule of eating and stick to it, just like you would stick to a schedule at your job. **A busy schedule is not an excuse to not eat or to make poor food choices; it just requires a little planning.** If you think you might be busy at a time when you normally eat, keep things like granola bars, cereal, dried fruit, nuts, or beef jerky with you. I don't go anywhere for long periods of time without having water and a snack with me. Pack lunches at night before you go to work, or freeze meal-sized portions of food on the weekend for the week ahead. It may feel like a pain in the butt while you're doing it, but it pays off big time later. It's nice to be able to just pull something out of your bag and eat it, instead of stressing out about what you're going to have. Also **make a list of healthy meal items you can grab at the grocery store or cafeteria just in case you forget or don't have time to pack a lunch.** Life happens; be prepared for it.

Commit to your meal plan by using a food journal. Your journal can be as simple as one of those 17 cent notebooks that are always on sale before the school year starts, or a word document on your phone or other electronic device that you keep with you (Don't just use one of those calorie counting apps—your goal is to *not* be counting calories anymore!). In your journal, write down your meal plan for the day and then record what you actually eat, including portion size and the times when you eat it. Also include how you feel physically and emotionally both before and after you eat. Doing so will help you learn a few things: 1) how to better understand your body's hunger and satiety signals, 2) how to differentiate physical from emotional hunger, and 3) which foods, times of day, or situations make eating more challenging for you.

Deb K., 43, from North Carolina said she referred to her journal any time she began to second-guess herself. She set aside a specific time to write in her journal each day and also made a habit of writing down questions she wanted to ask her therapist and dietitian when she showed them her journal. **Stay accountable by regularly showing your own food journal** to your dietitian, counselor, therapist, or someone else who will help keep you on track. It will be too easy for you to slip back into old ways if you don't have that accountability.

Remember that food is your medicine. It's only by letting go of your fears and actually *eating* that you will be able to heal. Your meal plan is your prescription for both physical health and emotional wellness. Like most people, Jessica, 29, from Texas, wasn't able to make any progress in her recovery until she actually began nourishing herself:

> *"I was so far gone mentally that it was pretty impossible to get any sense of authentic recovery without the proper nutrition and cessation of disordered behaviors. After about a month of proper nourishment, I was ready to take on the emotional lifestyle changes necessary to recover. I began to see that even though my eating disorder was not by choice, I could choose not to have one anymore."*

Let go of the guilt that may come with normal eating for you, because **you deserve to eat.** You're an amazing person with all kinds of incredible abilities, even if you don't recognize them in yourself right now. With continued effort toward recovery, you will discover and develop your abilities, identify your real aspirations in life, and begin figuring out how to make your dreams a reality (Refer back to Chapter Three for tips!). **Eating will give you the energy and concentration it takes to begin tackling your life goals:** You'll never know what kinds of remarkable things you're capable of doing until you start feeding your body and mind!

Make it a goal to let your healthy eating be an inspiration for others. There are probably plenty of people in your life who are trying to learn how to balance their own eating habits, and none of those crazy fad diet articles or advertisements are helping them, either. Try to upcycle your attitude about eating into one that can serve as a good example for others.

Stay flexible when life throws you a curveball. Use your meal plan to pack your lunches for the week, but don't let a packed lunch keep you from going out with your friends to the local café from time to time when the opportunity arises. The packed lunch will still be there and ready for you tomorrow. Also see Chapter Seven for more tips on specific challenging eating situations, like going out to eat at restaurants.

Remember that it's normal to feel a little bloated, puffy, or "yucky" while you're still getting used to your meal plan. Much of the reason I began to restrict food during my early, misguided attempts to recover from bulimia was because my metabolism was so sluggish as a result of what I'd been doing to my body. I was uncomfortable with the amount of extra water weight I seemed to be carrying, and didn't realize that my body would have started functioning normally much more quickly if I'd just kept eating like I was supposed to. The thing is, after your body has been in a state of starvation and malnutrition, it naturally needs a little time to regulate itself again. **Even though you might feel a little "full" before or during some meals, you still need to finish your food according to your plan.** As long as you stick with your plan and **visit your physician regularly to make sure everything is on track,** your body will adjust, your metabolism will improve, and you'll feel a whole lot better both inside and out. Those yucky feelings will go away.

Don't worry if you seem to be hungry all the time. Extreme hunger can occur after a period of malnourishment, because your body wants to get every little nutrient it can. There were times in my recovery when I felt like I could have just kept eating and eating and eating, until there was no food left in my house. That feeling went away once my body realized I wasn't starving anymore. Your hunger levels will stabilize too.

Keep paying attention to your emotions, and keep practicing healthy coping methods. If you're feeling extra yucky, try one of the activities on your "Alternative Activity" list from Chapter One, or call a friend to visit. The best thing you can do is get your mind off it.

Don't fall into the trap of always comparing what you're eating to others. Although the healthy people in your life can be great examples, don't stray from your meal plan based on what others are eating. If your friend is picking at a salad at lunch, it's not a reason for you to not finish your own food. Don't feel like you need to match your brother slice for slice when you go out for pizza. Unless you've spent every moment of every day with someone for a couple of weeks, there's no way for you to know exactly what they've been fueling their bodies with. Also, even if some of the people around you don't have eating disorders per se, they might not exactly be the best examples of healthy eating. There are a lot of people who overeat, make poor nutritional choices, or restrict on a regular basis. Don't let other people's choices derail *your* plans.

Try to pick healthy foods, but don't obsess over labels. Although some of the information on them can be helpful, your goal is to develop eating habits that are a natural, unobtrusive part of your life. You shouldn't feel the need to dig through the garbage at the next party you attend so you can check the packages the appetizers came out of. As long as you're following a basic meal plan, you'll be able to include moderate amounts of whatever you want in your diet.

Prevent yourself from getting overwhelmed: Besides breaking things up into smaller steps (interventions) like mentioned earlier in this chapter, when it comes to eating, try to just take each meal as it comes, rather than thinking about your whole day (or week) of food. But do plan ahead when it comes to *buying* that food: Jennifer, 30, from Missouri said it helps to **go grocery shopping at non-peak times** and **make a list before you go.** This will help you prevent a lot of anxiety and be able to make the right purchases.

Everything gets easier with time. Nicole Geddie, 24, from New Mexico remembers the first time she went to a grocery store alone, without feeling overwhelmed:

> *"I was so used to massive amounts of anxiety, tears even...I'd either end up piling a bunch of binge food in my basket...or a bunch of lettuce and celery, swearing I'd never eat another calorie again...or on occasion, my anxiety would reach the point that pushed me right out the door, empty-handed. I can't imagine how I must have looked to other shoppers. But I have a clear memory of that other grocery trip, when I felt calm, collected, and focused. I was pretty fresh out of the hospital at that point, and it was mind-blowing to me to experience this in such a different way! I called my mom on the phone just to tell her I wasn't overwhelmed! It was a very encouraging moment."*

Don't be shy about using your family and friends when you need to talk, or just need a hug or a hand to hold; that's what they're for. Be sure to **eat with other people as much as possible**, both for the emotional lift that comes from social interaction and the accountability that comes with having other people at the table with you. Make a conscious effort to distract yourself and *enhance* your relationships, by engaging in conversation with those around you: Those relationships are so much more important and fulfilling than anything on your plate!

Don't fall into the trap of counting calories. I did this for years, with the excuse that it was helping me make sure I didn't under-eat. The problem was that it was continuing to keep me hyper-focused on everything I ate. I couldn't just go out for lunch and figure out what a healthy-sized portion of anything was for me, because I was too busy calculating (and recalculating) all of the numbers for every little component of every meal I was considering in my head. Needless to say, I wasn't exactly present in any conversations, either! You don't need to be obsessive about everything you put in your mouth, as long as you're keeping a general log in your food diary so you can see patterns in what you're eating. A general log is enough to help you and the professionals you're working with identify whether or not you're getting the nutrition you need.

Don't eat directly out of containers, because that will make it harder for you to listen to your body and learn portion sizes. Instead, decide how much you're going to eat, and put that amount on a plate or in a bowl (again, you can learn more about portion sizes from your dietitian or on the U.S. Department of Agriculture website mentioned earlier). Then sit down at a table with it. Do your best to push away any of those negative thoughts you might have rushing at you—they can't sidetrack you if you don't listen to them!

Pay attention to the speed at which you eat: If you're the type of person who might end up restricting, try to eat at a normal pace, without dwelling on what you're doing. If you're feeling really anxious, flip through a magazine, watch some television, or make a list of things you want to do later. If you have the tendency to binge, be sure to take your time while you eat so that you're paying attention to each bite. Be mindful of the texture and flavor of the food, and remind yourself that you *will* be able to feel satisfied after eating the proper amount of it. Set down your silverware after you've finished eating, and brush your teeth if you can. Then put the food and any leftovers out of your mind: It will still be there tomorrow if you want a little more, and you're going to feel a whole lot more satisfied and comfortable knowing you've had the right-sized portion.

Have activities planned for after dinner, so you're not as likely to dwell on what you've just eaten. Put together a jigsaw puzzle, or take a leisurely walk outside. Refer to your "Alternative Activity" list from Chapter One for plenty of other ideas. If you find that you're still hungry 15 or 20 minutes later, find something to eat that you feel comfortable with, and measure out a portion of it again. Just make sure you have someone supportive with you if you're feeling a little apprehensive about it.

Then, just do your best to find things to do that will relax you. Talk with your friends and family, or spend some time writing in your journal.

Cheryl Kerrigan, 41, from Massachusetts, said meditation and yoga helped her deal with some of the uncomfortable feelings she experienced while adjusting to her meal plan:

> *"A deep breath can go a long way in getting your mind and body to come together. When I concentrate on my breath, my anxiety lessens and my body regulates itself into a calm state. In that calm state, my mind slows down and I am able to hear recovery and know that the uncomfortable feelings will pass…It's only short-term until your body learns where to rest and realizes you won't betray it again."*

Pay attention to how your body is feeling before, during, and after eating. If you feel a little (or a lot!) tense, concentrate on relaxing both your muscles and your breath. Remind yourself that what you are eating is healing your body and your mind.

Practice learning the difference between physical and emotional hunger: Physical hunger is usually more gradual, although it can take some practice to recognize some of the symptoms that are a little more subtle than a growling stomach! You might feel weak, tired, or lightheaded. You may notice that you're losing your concentration a little or becoming more irritable.

Emotional hunger can happen more suddenly. Maybe you notice yourself wanting to eat as soon as you start thinking about a big project that's due at work, or even after you receive some good news. Your hunger might be related to a specific comfort food, like potato chips or cookies, and you may still feel hungry even after you've been eating for awhile.

If you're physically hungry you might consider eating a wider variety of things than you would if you were emotionally hungry. A turkey sandwich might sound just as good as macaroni and cheese. As long as you're feeding yourself properly, physical hunger goes away shortly after you begin eating.

You won't always have to use a meal plan. Once you learn to identify and respond to your physical and emotional hunger signals, you'll begin the transition to intuitive eating. You might find yourself trying new foods, and eating at different times without even thinking about it. I've noticed that when I go on vacation and end up eating more fried foods and sweets than normal, I really do find myself craving the fresh fruits and vegetables my body needs.

Remember that your body is intelligent. If you're paying attention, you'll know what to eat. Your metabolism will stay healthy as long as you're eating healthily, and you won't end up bingeing on food if you're staying mindful and not depriving yourself. As long as you do all these things, **your body will settle at its "happy weight,"** where you feel best physically and emotionally. Alethia, 26, from Arizona, said that now that she's eating normally, her weight has stayed consistent even after 12 years of having an eating disorder and treating her body poorly:

> *"I learned to trust my body, and now it trusts me. For the last two years my bodyweight hasn't changed more than the normal five pounds it naturally fluctuates for women (depending on water, the time of the month, etc). My weight has stayed consistent without me weighing myself and then trying to adjust what I eat to that number. Some days I eat super-healthy, and other days I pig out—and my body deals with it. It trusts me now, and so my weight isn't really affected by those days when I eat a lot more."*

Brittany, 26, from Maryland, said that although she thought she'd gain a lot of weight once she stopped purging, it turned out to be actually quite the opposite:

> *"Now that I eat a healthy diet, it is much easier to maintain a healthy weight, compared to when I binged and purged on a regular basis. I can actually eat three meals a day plus snacks and not gain weight. I can eat foods that were previously forbidden, such as cake or ice cream and not gain weight. This wasn't easy for me to realize. It can be very difficult at first, because as you eat more, your body will naturally start to gain weight in order to reach a healthy weight. I never believed my body had a 'set point' for my weight, but now I firmly believe that is true. As you start eating more, your metabolism starts to increase as well—so you don't gain weight forever. Eventually when your body is back to a healthy weight, you will start to maintain your weight even when you are eating larger amounts than you are used to."*

It's amazing how great your body is at telling you what it needs; you just have to listen.

Below are your journal questions, followed by this chapter's family segment and Q & A section:

Journal Questions

1. How did I naturally eat as a child? How can I learn from that?

2. How am I feeling about the way I'm eating now? What do I need to work on? What are some specific steps I can take to improve my diet?

3. What are some positive things I'm hoping to experience as I begin to nourish myself better?

4. What are the most difficult physical effects I'm experiencing right now? Why might they be happening? What can I do to make myself feel more comfortable?

Tips for Friends & Family

Help me stay relaxed around mealtime.

The time immediately before, during, and after a meal can be particularly stressful for your loved one. Be there for support and keep him or her engaged in conversation; however, try not to talk about sensitive topics at this time. For a period of time, those in recovery from anorexia may be helped by having board games or crossword puzzles available to help them get their mind off of the food in front of them, while those recovering from bulimia or binge eating disorder do better by staying mindful of what they're eating. Ask your loved one what will help him or her the most.

Help me stay on track.

Denial and complacency can be tough to beat no matter what issue you're dealing with, let alone an eating disorder. Tara, 29, from Michigan said it's important to "bring us back to reality, no matter how stubborn we are, and remind us that a cup of cereal is not the gigantic breakfast that we think it is."

Cheryl Kerrigan, 41, from Massachusetts also suggested family members support their loved ones by offering to grocery shop and cook meals with them—two tasks that can be anxiety-inducing for someone in recovery.

Questions Friends & Family Should Ask

1. How are you feeling about your meal plan?

2. What can we do to make it easier for you to follow your meal plan?

3. How can we make mealtime more pleasant?

Journal Questions for Friends & Family

1. What questions do I have about healthy eating?

2. How can I be supportive of my loved one's meal plan?

3. How can I be a positive example?

Q & A with Barbara Truitt, RD, LD/N

Q: What kinds of physical effects might I experience as I learn to eat more normally?

A: When you restrict or purge, your cells become dehydrated and "shriveled;" once you begin to eat and/or stop purging, the cells hold on to the water for a longer time than usual in order to keep themselves "puffed up." This puffing up is felt as water weight.

It is important to know that once the eating and/or ceasing of purging is more regular, the cells realize this and release the added water slowly. Many people become frightened when they feel the water weight. It can be very difficult to convince a person in an "eating disorder" state that this water weight is temporary. When it is not realized, the restricting or purging cycle begins.

Q: How can I deal with some of the uncomfortable physical effects of a normal meal plan?

A: An eating disorder is going to cause those feelings—however, antacids and other over-the-counter medicines can only aggravate the condition, which will prolong the irritation. The difficulties are the esophagus, stomach, and bowel "healing themselves."

Avoid highly-acidic foods in the beginning of "normal eating," such as pickles, vinegar, and vinegar-based dressings, barbecue sauce, tomato juice, and tomato sauce. Slowly work these foods back into the diet within six to nine months.

Q: How can I find a dietitian who will understand my circumstances?

A: I recommend first going to support groups, where someone may share the name of their Registered Dietitian with you. Otherwise, go to http://www.eatright.org and click in the upper right hand corner to find a nutrition professional. This is a nationwide website.

Q: How can I form a good relationship with my dietitian?

A: Be honest with your nutritionist. It is frustrating if a client relapses once or twice between visits and doesn't come clean. **You may relapse, and it is the job of your therapist and nutritionist to help you reduce the number of relapses.**

Don't let someone who may have had a bad experience with a nutritionist talk you into thinking all nutritionists are bad. There are many people out there who want to help you—please know that they want to see you recover!

Q: Can't I just figure out what I'm supposed to be eating on my own?

A: You are playing with danger. You run a high risk of either overeating, which could lead to a purge, or a high risk of not meeting your nutritional needs. Either way, by trying to "guess" or "figure out" on your own, it can start a cycle.

Q: What are the biggest misconceptions people with eating disorders have about nutrition?

A: People in recovery often believe that food contains more fat and calories than it really does. A common comment about bread is: "It will turn to cement in my stomach." Those with eating disorders do not see that the food is nourishing the body to keep glucose going to the brain, building muscles, and feeding our vital organs, especially the kidneys and heart.

Q: How do the needs of clients with anorexia and bulimia compare?

A: Both actually need to keep the same "nutrition concept" in mind: They must realize that there are many nutrients that must be consumed to maintain life and that the nutrients must be allowed to be absorbed and digested. Restricting and purging both may lead to stunted growth and interfere with bone, muscle, and organ development. The end result of anorexia or bulimia left untreated is, ultimately, heart failure.

Q: How important is structure in meal planning? How structured—or not—should it be? Is it different from person to person?

A: Meal planning should always be done on an individual basis. Asking some people to measure their food will not cause them to feel triggered, while for others it will. Each meal plan is different, and the nutritional value varies based on many factors: Current weight, ideal bodyweight, age, gender, and activity level.

Q: How do you help your clients feel more comfortable while learning to eat more normally?

A: It is important to remember that everyone is in a different place in their disorder. However, I like to conduct MST (Mealtime Support Therapy) with clients, either one-on-one or in a group. I find it usually works better for everyone when MST is conducted in a group. MST helps everyone provide support to each other and get through a meal without anxiety.

Mealtime Support Therapy is where people who are in treatment for eating disorders, eat a meal with a dietitian and sometimes a therapist as well. Feelings, urges to binge, and urges to restrict or purge can be spoken out loud. The dietitian, therapist, and other group members can offer support and help provide coping skills to use to get through the meal. The dietitian and therapist also have rules; they will give a specific time period in which the meal is to be eaten, they will remind you to slow down if you are eating too fast, and they will remind you to eat a little faster if someone is struggling. When offered on a regular basis, it can guarantee this person will eat a certain number of meals.

If MST is not offered in your area, you can find a friend or an eating disorder sponsor to join you during your most difficult meals. Have them openly call you out if you are cutting food too small, or performing other eating rituals. Tell them coping skills that work for you, so if needed, they can remind you of them when the meal becomes difficult.

Q: How can I get more protein?

A: Here are some things you can try:

1. Add two teaspoons of dry milk powder to hot chocolate, smoothies, soup, mashed potatoes, pudding, yogurt, scrambled eggs, and hot cereal.
2. Sprinkle shredded cheese or parmesan cheese on soups, pasta, chicken, and rice.
3. Purchase protein-enriched food products (milk, cereal, margarine, etc.).
4. Add nuts to yogurt or cereal.
5. Use milk in place of water when making mashed potatoes, soup, or hot cereal.
6. Use yogurt for dipping vegetables.

Barbara Truitt's Quick, Healthy Recipes for All Meal Plans

Make-Your-Own Trail Mix
(Makes 10 Servings)

1 cup of a high fiber cereal (8 grams per serving or more)
1 cup of any cold cereal
1 cup of dried fruit with raisins (you can use yogurt-covered raisins)
¾ cup of any kind of nut
½ cup sunflower or pumpkin seeds
3 crumbled cereal bars of your choice

Mix all ingredients into one bowl, then separate into 10-12 sandwich-sized baggies. Keep these on hand for snacks, doctors' appointments, or for short road trips.

Breakfast Smoothie
(Makes One Serving)

½ cup plain or vanilla yogurt
½ cup ice
½ cup any fresh or frozen fruit
2 teaspoons dry milk powder
1 teaspoon wheat germ
1 tablespoon flavored granola

Pour all ingredients into a blender and mix to your preferred consistency.

Snack Smoothie
(Makes One Serving)

½ cup plain or vanilla yogurt
½ cup ice
¼ cup fresh or frozen fruit

Pour all ingredients into a blender and mix to your favorite consistency.

Make-Your-Own Egg Muffin
(Makes One Serving)

1 toasted wholegrain English muffin, with margarine on both sides*
2 scrambled egg whites

2 slices tomato
2 slices onion

Assemble all cooked ingredients on the toasted bread.

**One 10-inch wholegrain wrap can be substituted for the English muffin (omit margarine).*

Q & A with Doris Smeltzer

Q: What do I do if someone I love is trying to be the "food police" for me, or control any of my other behaviors now that they know about my disorder?

A: Knowledge is sometimes the best antidote to less than helpful responses. I would encourage my loved ones to speak to my treatment team members (skilled therapist, dietitian, physician, etc.) about who is responsible for what when it comes to your specific healing process. A great resource for parents is Duke University's manual, *Off the C.U.F.F.* (to order: http://bit.ly/VNCXEW). Other informative resources can be found on the NEDA website: http://www.nationaleatingdisorders.org/family-and-friends; or check out our "Eating Disorders Information" link for book suggestions and additional helpful websites: http://andreasvoice.org/fighting-eating-disorders. Encouraging loved ones to learn all they can about eating disorders can help them better understand how they can support and advocate for your healing, and maintain balance and sanity in the process.

Q & A with Carolyn Costin, MFT, M.ED., and Keesha Broome, M.A., MFT

Q: What does "refeeding" mean?

A: Refeeding is a term used to describe the process of reintroducing food and monitoring the physical implications, known as refeeding syndrome. Generally speaking, it is the severely-emaciated, malnourished patient with prolonged starvation who is at risk for refeeding syndrome.

It is comforting to know that the refeeding process takes time, but also that when taken care of, the body will respond appropriately. The motto for adding calories is to start low and go slow. This is due to the fact that in the past, many people were refed too fast and thus had several problems because the body has to adapt to digesting and metabolizing food. If not done properly, electrolytes can be thrown out of balance and edema and serious heart problems can occur. But if you work with a professional who knows eating disorders and how to establish a refeeding protocol, it can be done safely.

Q: How will I know when I'm ready to just eat intuitively?

A: We believe that it is important to begin experimenting with intuitive eating while working with a dietitian, if possible, so that you have the necessary support. Regularly adding some variety to your meal plan is one way to add a more intuitive approach to your recovery. Some ways to do this are choosing different snacks every day or challenging yourself to try one new food. You can also try other small steps such as having a dinner out that is not on your meal plan and then work up to a day off your meal plan and then a weekend.

With the help of a dietitian or therapist, you can also start experimenting with eating different percentages of meals to test physical hunger and fullness. For example, eat to the point of fullness at dinner, rather than just eating all that's on your plate because your meal plan says to. It is important to keep a journal when doing this so that you can check in with yourself to gauge physical and emotional feelings after each meal. This helps you to figure out whether or not you are eating according to your body, or to your emotions.

It's good to have an objective source to give you feedback and help you assess your readiness to let go of a structured meal plan. There are also several books that can be useful in working towards this goal. Once you have challenged yourself with these things and discussed your progress with your dietitian and/or treatment team, you can better evaluate your ability to eat more intuitively. It is important to note that intuitive eating is more difficult if you have not reached your natural weight, because you usually have to eat more than you feel like eating to gain weight. It is hard when you are undernourished and fearful of weight gain to really tune to your body's feelings of hunger and fullness.

7 Order Something New: Facing "food fears" and tough eating situations

"Old habits cannot be thrown out the upstairs window. They must be coaxed down the stairs one step at a time."

–Mark Twain

What's the difference between someone in recovery and someone who's fully recovered? Someone who is recovered isn't afraid of food—any kind of it. Before my own transition from bulimia to anorexia, I had had the best intentions of eating as healthily as possible. Unfortunately, I was plagued with fears that certain foods might just trigger me to overeat and possibly even purge again. My concerns about eating normally intensified after I began reading about the idea of "clean eating" in some of my fitness magazines. If you're not familiar with the concept, clean eating involves focusing on unpackaged, unprocessed foods that are as close to their natural state as possible, including whole grains, proteins, fruits and vegetables, and healthy fats. It also typically involves eating small meals more frequently throughout the day, instead of the standard three meals and snacks.

The principles behind clean eating are wonderful, because you still include all of the main food groups and you're actually encouraged to *eat.* So what was my problem? It's not the best idea for someone who's trying to learn how to *not* be restrictive to be memorizing another list of "good" and "bad" foods. For years, I treated certain foods almost like they were poisonous. I wouldn't touch a piece of white bread, and only allowed myself nibbles of anything that came in bags or boxes, for fear that they'd turn me into some overweight, massively unhealthy person. I took the principles behind clean eating to the point where I allowed my eating habits to interfere with my life. I couldn't eat without analyzing the nutritional content of everything on my plate, and I continued to do everything possible to avoid eating with other people, because I knew there would be no way for me to control what we ate or how it was prepared.

Again, I'm not saying that clean eating in itself is a bad thing—it just wasn't a good idea for someone like me at that time to be keeping "rules" about what I could and couldn't eat. I'm sure there are plenty of people who follow this way of eating and still maintain a healthy mindset, but it can be much more challenging for those who are early in their recovery. The more I told myself I couldn't have certain things, the more I craved them. I still remember a time a few years ago when someone dropped a chunk of chocolate chip cookie on an old rug outside my apartment, and all I could think about was how much I would have loved to just eat it—dirty or not. There were other times when I'd hungrily eye the chunks of pasta, partial leftover sandwiches, and other uneaten food I'd see in the trash after my family threw it away. The more I outlawed certain foods, the more my cravings for them grew, and the more I was afraid of their "power" over me.

Even though clean eating is a wonderful way to eat, a healthy and happy life will always include a balanced variety of foods. You can make most of your food choices based on what's best for your body, but also allow yourself treats every once in awhile, too, so you stay emotionally healthy and don't miss out on any fun times with friends and family that might involve food. Healthy diets include sometimes having things just because they taste good, like cake at a birthday party, or a sundae cone from the ice cream truck on a really hot day.

Despite everything I believed a few years ago, eating a piece of white bread instead of 100% whole wheat isn't going to make you gain weight or make your fat cells swell up and burst into a wave of cellulite across your thighs. The whole wheat bread does have more fiber, which can help you feel more satiated, but eating it instead of the white isn't in itself going to make a difference in the physical appearance of your body. I still pay attention to what I eat because it does have an impact on my health, mood, and energy levels. However, there's no such thing as a "never" food for me anymore—if I want something, I have some of it. Because of that, I don't get crazy, out of control cravings, and I feel satisfied when I eat. I have fun at social gatherings, instead of making up excuses to get out of going to them. I'm at peace, both with my body and in my daily life.

This chapter is filled with tips to help you overcome some of the food fears that are keeping you from living your best life. Later on you'll also find tips on how you can relax and eat well despite some common challenging eating situations, like going out to restaurants, handling holiday meals, eating with family members, and more.

Let's get started!

Conquer "Food Fears"

Have you ever told someone you were lactose intolerant as an excuse not to eat ice cream, or that you stay away from pizza because it always makes you break out? Ever pass up on a freshly-baked cinnamon roll after claiming to be allergic to gluten, or turned down a slice of caramel apple pie because you "just don't like it?" **Be honest with yourself** about your reasons for avoiding certain foods. Do you really not like them? Are you genuinely allergic to them, or are you just afraid to eat them?

If you suspect you have a legitimate allergy or intolerance related to a certain type of food, don't just tell people you're not supposed to eat it, without any basis for that claim; visit your physician and find out what's actually going on with your body. You'll be able to manage your food issues and your health much better once you're properly educated about them.

However, if you're avoiding certain foods because of any fears you may have about them, try to **analyze your fear:** Where is that fear coming from? Where did you get the idea that you "can't" or "shouldn't" have that food? **Reframe your feelings** by recognizing that many of the negative ideas you have about certain foods may be the result of disordered thoughts, or even just incorrect information you've gotten from random magazines or other people. Remind yourself that a healthy diet and a happy life include a balance of all kinds of foods. Restriction and fear don't make anyone healthy or happy!

Put your fears into perspective. Allie, 23, from Pennsylvania noted some interesting differences between a friend's and her own food fears:

> *"One of my friends was afraid of fatty foods but had no problem eating carbohydrates. She could go through an entire bag of candy corn in one sitting and not feel guilty, but if she had peanut butter crackers or a high-fat salad dressing, she would get horrible anxiety and usually end up purging. I, on the other hand, would have horrible feelings about myself and my body after eating something like candy corn, but peanut butter crackers didn't bother me much at all. Once you see something like that, it makes you realize how irrational your mind can be. If one person is afraid of something you're not afraid of, and you're afraid of something they're not, where is the sense in that?"*

Challenge your fears by confronting them. Even if it's the last thing in the world you want to do, the only way to overcome your fears is by actually eating the food you've been avoiding. Rayna, 26, from Ohio, shared how her attitude has changed ever since she learned to challenge her food fears:

> *"One of the best things I've rediscovered since recovering from my eating disorder? French fries. Especially the super-crunchy, salty ones. Garlic fries. Sweet potato fries. McDonald's fries. They're all wonderful. Sadly, however, I spent years denying my love of french fries to both others and myself. I stopped ordering them at restaurants, telling myself that I couldn't possibly consume all those calories and fat. I was quite certain I would instantly see the results of this crime on my hips and*

stomach. And so I slowly became convinced that not only did I not need (or deserve) french fries, I didn't like them. I spent years substituting fruit and cottage cheese and vegetables when asked what I'd like at restaurants: French fries? Gross! Who would want all that grease? No thank you, Ma'am. I'll have the peas.

"While in treatment, I was presented with 'challenge foods,' items that most individuals with eating disorders find difficult to eat, usually due to their nutritional status. One time french fries were presented as the challenge food and I thought I might die. Right there. Fall out of my chair and die. My reaction to this item was a clue to me. Was I so fearful because it was something I didn't like the taste of? Or was it something else? Pushing through the exercise and eating the fries for the first time I had them in several years, I realized that they weren't so disgusting. They might even be…good. In the weeks and months that followed I began to push myself to order fries while out to lunch and dinner—not all the time, but occasionally. I quickly came to remember my fondness for this classic American delicacy, but now, my new skills allowed me to stop when I was full. I realized that my fear of not being able to control my desire for this food had warped into a steadfastly held belief that it was something I didn't like. I realized just how powerful our minds could be at that point, and how I needed to continue challenging myself and beginning to practice trusting myself with my favorite foods. And now? I eat french fries at least once a week, and I love them. Especially the super-crunchy, salty ones."

Don't deny yourself the opportunity to rediscover your own favorite foods. They're a wonderful part of life! **Plan your own food challenge, and figure out what it will look like *before* you do it. Ask yourself these questions as a guide:**

1. What food are you going to eat? Pizza? Ice cream? Cookies? As far as your specific challenge goes, **it's okay to start small**—you don't have to eat a whole double cheeseburger if you haven't eaten anything but tofu in years. Start with a few bites of a plain burger for your first challenge, then half of it for your second, and then have the whole burger along with a side salad for a third challenge.

2. Where are you going to eat it? At a restaurant, picnic in the park, birthday party? **Consider completing your challenge somewhere other than your home**, where you might feel more compelled to go back to old bad habits. Going somewhere you've never gone before may also be very helpful: A change of scenery can make you *feel* like a different person who is more capable of making positive choices. If you have some social anxiety, you may consider doing your first challenge or two at home, *as long as you are not alone*, and as long as future challenges prepare you to begin feeling more comfortable eating around other people (See the next section for more tips on social eating situations).

3. Who will be with you? Your mom or dad? A friend? Your counselor? **Make sure you have someone supportive with you** to talk to and get reassurance from while you're eating. This isn't optional; it's required.

4. What will you do after your challenge? Go for a walk, go window shopping, go to a movie, take an art class? **Have something fun planned for after your challenge** so you're not dwelling on what you've just eaten. Focus on getting out and experiencing life, instead of staying stuck in your head and worrying about food!

Above all, just **try to relax** as much as possible and **plan to keep including your challenge foods regularly in your meal plan** until you feel more comfortable eating them. You'll see that you can eat all those things you're craving, *without* them causing any freakish metamorphoses in your body. You can have one of your grandma's special raisin cinnamon rolls for breakfast sometimes, just like the rest of your family. You can eat pizza and ice cream, and when there's a birthday celebration at work, you don't have to be the only one running in the *opposite* direction of the cake. **Don't listen to your eating disorder; listen to your heart.**

Normal, healthy eating also includes feeling comfortable in social food situations. As I said earlier, I used to do everything I could to avoid eating meals with other people. Besides not being able to control what was served, I was always a little worried everyone else would be watching me the whole time I ate. However, it wasn't until I learned to let go of some of my food "quirks" and start eating with other people that I began to have real friends again, and actually realize how much I preferred them to any of my old obsessive dining rituals. If I hadn't learned to eat with other people, I would still be the same lonely, insecure person that I was just a few years ago. My husband and I wouldn't have been able to make the very special connection we made on our first date if I'd just been staring down at my plate the whole time, anxiously counting each piece of chicken in my pasta at the Italian restaurant he suggested we go to—or even worse, if I'd just decided not to go. After all, pasta most certainly was *not* on my former "good" list of foods!

Because I went on that first date, and because I was more interested in the connection we were making than what was on my plate, our first few hours together were actually pretty amazing: We talked about our families and our values, and some of our life experiences. We laughed about silly and ridiculous things. We had such a great time on our dinner date that we extended it by driving all around town looking at Christmas lights, and then just looking for any random store still open at 10 p.m. on a Monday night so we could spend more time together, under the guise of getting some Christmas shopping done. That dinner date truly ended up becoming the wonderful beginning to one of the most cherished and rewarding relationships I ever could have imagined. I'm so glad I didn't stay home with a bowl of oatmeal that night!

Challenge yourself to really get out of your comfort zone, stop depriving yourself, and give yourself an active and *complete* social life. Here's how you can learn to eat with other people, and actually start to *enjoy* it:

Social Eating (without Anxiety)

As much as you might hate to hear this, the first step to feeling more comfortable on outings with other people is to **face your fears.** Say yes the next time someone asks you to go out for dinner, or **invite a supportive friend or family member to go to a restaurant with you to practice first.** Go to a restaurant you feel comfortable with for the first couple of times, and talk through any tough feelings you experience.

Don't forget to **eat moderately throughout the day,** so your hunger levels are more stable when you do go out. Stick to your meal plan. As tempting as it may be to try to restrict your food beforehand, you're not nearly as likely to be able to make good choices if you're ravenously hungry by the time you get there. Following your plan will also help you avoid some of the anxiety that comes with overthinking or trying to alter your eating habits before going out.

Don't make comparisons between what and how much you and others are eating. A lot of people tend to do this sometimes, but it's counterproductive because each person's needs are very different from anyone else's. What one person eats at a single restaurant meal may not be anything like what a well-rounded meal should look like for you. **Make choices based on what you need,** and not on what anyone else is doing. When you're ordering, try to pick a balanced meal with a mix of protein, carbohydrates, fiber, and some healthy fat. If you're at a party or buffet, take a quick walk around the food tables to see what's being offered, and then take a moment to think about which foods you would like to have. If you're feeling overwhelmed by endless food options, keep in mind that you don't have to eat or even try everything. Keep it balanced, and if there's something there that you absolutely love, go ahead and take a little bit of it—that's what normal eating is!

Once you have your food, eat at a reasonable pace; be mindful not to eat too quickly if you have problems with bingeing, and not too slowly if you tend to restrict. Also be wary of the effects certain drinks may have on you: Is the caffeine in your soda going to make you feel more anxious? Will the alcohol in your cocktail hinder your resolve to stick to your recovery? Remember to stay balanced!

As tough as it may be, **don't worry that everyone else might be**

watching what you're eating. As long as you're not partaking in any weird food rituals, chances are they won't be. They have their own plates and probably have plenty of their own thoughts and worries up in their heads. They might ask a question or two about what you're eating and how it tastes simply because people are curious—but as long as you don't act awkward about what you're eating, they probably won't give it a second thought either. If anyone *does* keep asking questions or seem to be overly interested in what you're eating, it may be because they have some food (or other) issues of their own. Just do your best to brush it off, and remind them that they have food on their own plate to worry about. Make light of it if you can.

Above all, **stay calm and be confident in your food choices.** It's when you constantly second-guess everything you're eating that you set yourself up to start engaging in unhealthy eating habits. Even if you don't eat exactly how you plan to, it's just one meal and one meal is not going to affect you. Don't dwell on it.

Nicole Geddie, 24, from New Mexico, said that isolating herself from other people because of her anxiety, only made things worse for her:

> *"It started chipping at my relationships, and dragged me deeper into my eating disorder...and the deeper you allow yourself to go, the harder it is to climb back out again. You have to treat those situations like exposures: In treatment I had to learn how to sit with my binge foods without bingeing, how to walk through 'binge' aisles of the grocery store without buying food, and how to eat in restaurants without purging. It's the same for learning to eat with other people. When you force yourself to tolerate the anxiety and the discomfort, you realize you ARE capable of doing it, and over time, it gets easier."*

Are you still pretty nervous about eating with other people? Take your attention away from the food itself, and **focus on the experience and your relationships.** Stay in the moment and stay active in the conversation. Don't let your worries make you miss out on the fun! Remember also that **sharing food is one of the oldest and most natural ways to bond and build relationships with other people.** Since positive relationships are usually linked to greater feelings of satisfaction and happiness, it makes sense to start eating with other people more often.

That being said, eating with other people still might not be the easiest thing in the world for you at first. If you're feeling pretty apprehensive, **prepare yourself to stay engaged in conversation by having discussion topics ready before you go out.** Keep a few questions in your mind to ask, or even write some down in a little notepad or on notecards in your bag. Ask your friends what the best thing was that happened to them this week, what new TV shows they've been getting into, if they've learned anything new at work, or anything else you can think of. Having questions ready will help you enjoy your time and learn more about your company, instead of letting your worries run wild. If you do find yourself fighting off negative thoughts, **keep practicing the relaxation techniques that help you most,** like deep breathing or whatever else works for you. **Make a conscious effort to refocus your mind:** Think about how every bite is nurturing and healing your body and brain, and remind yourself that every time you eat with other people you'll just keep getting better at it.

Shannon, 22, from Texas, said she is happy she can now have conversations without constantly thinking about calories:

> *"Being able to be in the moment is huge. I have great memories of the year I recovered, like sharing a dessert with my mom on my birthday—I mean little things that others may not think much about. I have learned to appreciate feelings and memories, because really when I look back, it's not going to be how much I weighed that day or what foods I ate—it's going to be the people I was with, and the feelings I had, that I'm going to remember."*

There's nothing better than being able to actually enjoy food with other people, without having your head stuck in a cloud of worry. One of the most difficult times to do that is definitely during the holidays and at other special occasions, when it seems like everyone around you is even more food-obsessed than usual. So how do you navigate those office parties, family dinners, and other celebrations, without feeling anxious or overwhelmed?

Holiday & Other Special Occasion Eating

During the holidays there are tasty goodies everywhere, and every gathering usually includes enough food to feed three times as many guests as those actually present! Don't get overwhelmed by all the platters and trays of cookies and bars and candies that seem to magically appear by the minute at certain times of the year—it's all about balance. **You don't have to try everything at once,** and **you don't have to finish everything;** it's okay to just have a taste. **Holidays also shouldn't become justifications to go back to old unhealthy behaviors**, even if you think it's "just for one day." One day can easily turn into several days, and even a single day makes it immensely harder for you to stay on the right path. Don't restrict, and if you have the tendency to binge, be mindful and remember that you don't have to keep eating things once they're not tasting as good to you anymore.

When it comes to those holiday parties and dinners, a lot of the tips above will be helpful. But one of the nice things about those celebrations is that you can always **offer to bring a dish or two of something you like**

to eat. That way you know you'll always have some choices you feel comfortable with. Just don't use it as an excuse to stay in your same old food ruts. The holidays can be a wonderful time to **challenge yourself to try new things,** especially if you have the support of family and friends. Cheryl Kerrigan, 41, from Massachusetts said that as she got stronger in her recovery, she would challenge herself to eat what she craved, as well as try new things. She savored each bite, and allowed herself to have more if she wanted it. She found it helpful to **use affirmations to feel more relaxed:**

> *"Before I went to the party I would say out loud to myself, 'I am allowed to eat any food there; all food is okay to eat.' It was a positive mantra I used to help me go outside my comfort level...and it worked."*

Before you go to your next party, be ready with a couple of your own affirmations. Tell yourself how much better the experience is going to be as long as you don't worry about the food, and remind yourself that you're perfectly capable of making healthy choices. At the party, also **be mindful of where you're sitting or standing.** Instead of staying right next to the food table and staring at it after you fill your plate, go somewhere else and get involved in a conversation. **Keep in mind the reasons everyone is gathered there in the first place;** as amazing as the food may be, it's only a small part of the celebration. **Take a quick time out if you start to feel overwhelmed.** Go outside for a breath of fresh air, take a quick walk, or call someone you can talk to. Then get back to where the action is and try to enjoy the party!

Be mindful and stay balanced as much as possible, but remember that **it's okay if you eat a little more than you plan every once in awhile.** Your body is smart and can adjust to occasional extra treats.

If you find yourself receiving all kinds of tasty goodies as gifts at certain times during the year, spread the love by sharing some of it at your office, school, or in your neighborhood. If you *ever* find yourself left with any food you know might tempt you a little too much to binge or purge—even if Grandma gives you a great big care package of leftovers after your Thanksgiving meal—don't feel like you have to eat all of it. You can always vacuum-seal it or freeze it into some "just right" portions so you don't have to look at it, or give it away to your friends or your neighbors (especially those who have a little trouble in the kitchen!). Even if some of the food just ends up in the garbage bin outside, I promise that Grandma will never know. And besides—throwing a little bit of food away is a whole lot less wasteful than throwing away your recovery!

Protect yourself no matter what time of year it is. If you're feeling a little nervous at the idea of having a whole bunch of candy around your house before and after Halloween, don't be afraid to be the person who gives out toothbrushes or apples instead. Ask your sweetie for flowers or a teddy bear for Valentine's Day instead of a big box of chocolates.

If you're doing your own cooking or baking for a special occasion, invite someone else over to help you out. It'll help you stay accountable and you'll probably end up having a lot more fun. **If you're in charge of cooking a whole holiday meal, break it up into smaller tasks,** like Alethia, 26, from Arizona does:

> *"...cook a few foods, along with one challenging food, and do that until everything is made. And take breaks...Even people without eating disorders don't cook everything in one ginormous swoop—holiday meals can shake even the sanest of mind. Give yourself time and breaks."*

Ashley Devitt, 18, from Florida said she likes to focus on senses other than taste when she bakes:

> *"I try to enjoy the texture when kneading the cookie dough, or cherish the smell of the apple pie baking in the oven, or even put on some festive music to set a holiday mood in the kitchen. I've found that when I truly acknowledge and appreciate other sensory elements in the kitchen, besides taste, I do not even worry about the thought of bingeing."*

Allow yourself to taste what you're making without feeling guilty; all foods are good in moderation! Jan Lockert, 53, from Ohio remembers the first time she allowed herself to leave room for more flexibility in her meal plan:

> *"I had started dating a man I met through a dinner dating club. He liked to cook...One evening when I was at his place he decided that he wanted to bake a cake, so we did it together. When it had baked and was ready for icing, he opened a can of premade frosting, stuck a spoon in it, and held it out to my mouth. I didn't hesitate. I opened my mouth and took the bite of frosting. I surprised myself, and it made quite an impact on my own confidence for recovery. I had never allowed myself to 'taste' foods as I was cooking, or to add a spoonful of any food to my meal plan—especially something like frosting! That simple act was important to my recovery and my own self-confidence."*

Taste things, and don't give yourself the chance to feel overwhelmed: When you're done baking, seal the goodies in containers and put them somewhere you won't be looking at them all the time.

If spending time in the kitchen cooking and baking triggers you, **don't feel bad about buying something from the grocery store when you're asked to contribute to a potluck;** Alethia, 26, from Arizona also suggested picking something up and putting it in your own dish, like she does for work potlucks.

Above all, **remember to find ways for you and your family to keep the meaning of all those special days.** Have some fun taking part in old traditions, or start a few new ones: Make cute ornaments, sing carols, or volunteer together for the holidays. Carve pumpkins at Halloween, or go shopping at local thrift stores to create your very own unique costumes. Instead of just sitting around thinking about food all day long on Thanksgiving, get a few of your family members outside for a fun walk, a game of touch-football, or to shoot a few hoops. Another fun Thanksgiving activity is to give everyone slips of paper where they can write down the things they're most thankful for—they can be silly or serious things. When everyone is finished, put all of the slips into a hat or bowl. After dinner, have each person draw one slip out, read it, and try to guess who wrote it.

Have holiday-specific movie or game nights, or seasonal crafts-making parties with your friends. If you want to get everyone a little more involved, you can ask each person to bring their own movie, game, or craft project. If you're not such a creative person, go online or to your local library to find ideas for some games and crafts. On Valentine's Day you can make cute little cards for everyone you know, just like in grade school. You can find fun new ways to decorate eggs on Easter, or make colorful paper decorations for St. Patrick's Day or the Fourth of July. Don't you just love holidays?

Now, what if you're staying with family or others for longer than just a holiday meal? Here's how you can enjoy your visit without fret:

Family Visits

Although it can be hard for your family to hear, it's important to be truthful about any anxieties you may experience while you're at home. When I first began attempting to recover from bulimia, I tried to pretend I was perfectly comfortable around any kind of food I came across around the house. I didn't want to admit that I was actually terrified of some of the foods I found on the counter or in the cupboards. It can also be tough to go back to a place where you may have struggled a lot with your eating, both because of family dynamics and because of any old memories and feelings that may be brought up again. Let your family know what they can do to help ease your mind while you're with them. If you discuss your meal plan together, they'll at least have a general idea of what and how often you need to be eating. **Although it's important that you don't try to change or control your family's habits, being open with them will let them know how they can help make things a little easier for you.**

If there's a whole lot of food lying around, ask your family to help keep it out of sight so you won't be thinking about it all the time. **Let**

them know if there are times when you might feel triggered, like when you're tired or you know you're going to be alone for a period of time. **With your family you can figure out what kinds of things you can do to feel a little more secure:** Could you plan to go somewhere else for awhile? Could you call your loved ones if you start to feel a little uncomfortable? What are some healthy activities you can do?

Go grocery shopping. Although it's important that you try to eat all your meals with your family, it's also important to be prepared with some of your favorite snacks when you need to eat. After I started talking to my parents more honestly about some of my food issues, we went to the store together to stock up on things I felt good about eating, rather than me having to just try to fill up on whatever I could find in the house.

Make yourself at home. Depending on the length of your stay, ask your family if they'd be willing to designate a shelf in the pantry or a section of the refrigerator or freezer with the healthy snacks and foods you've incorporated into your meal plan. Make sure you keep a moderate amount of food there—not so much that you may feel tempted to binge, but enough so you know you won't run out, either.

If you find yourself surrounded by a whole bunch of food, remember that it *isn't* your sole responsibility to consume it so it doesn't "go to waste." Extra food can always go into the freezer for another time! Just the same, **don't let anxiety put you back into restriction mode.** Talk to someone in your family about how all that extra food is making you feel, or call a friend. Discuss what kinds of things you'd feel comfortable eating, based both on your meal plan and your tastes. That in itself should help you feel a little more at ease.

Consider portioning out food for yourself. Sometimes when I used to go home and see a whole pile of dinner rolls, I would set aside a couple of them for myself by putting them in a separate container. To me, looking at only those two rolls seemed more manageable than looking at the whole big pile and then either nervously picking them apart or eating more than I was comfortable with. Doing that helped me remember to just eat my own food at my own pace, without thinking about the rest of the pile and how it might get thrown out if no one ate it.

Help your family prepare meals that you all can enjoy. If your family loves to eat lots of fried, greasy food and you tend to stick to lighter fare, compromise and find some new recipes. Coat some chicken with egg, seasonings, and panko (Japanese) bread crumbs and bake it in the oven until it's nice and crispy. Make dessert smoothies out of frozen bananas, cocoa powder, pudding powder, and a little milk to thin it. There are lots of fun things out there to try once you start looking a little!

Connect in ways that are unrelated to food. **Remember to have a deck of cards or a fun board game handy for after dinner, or suggest something fun to do while you're at home and Mom is cooking up a**

storm. Food shouldn't be the focus!

Next are your journal questions, followed by this chapter's family section and Q & A segment.

Journal Questions

1. Are there any food groups I'm having trouble incorporating? Are there any foods I've told myself I "don't like," only because I'm afraid to eat them? What fears might I have related to some of these foods?

2. What steps will I take to help myself reincorporate some of the foods I'm afraid of? How can I make myself feel more comfortable while eating them? Who can support me?

3. How did I feel after a recent challenging meal? What did I do well? What areas might I need to work on (Ex: eating with more balance, not restricting or overeating, etc.)?

Tips for Friends & Family

Try to understand (even if you can't relate).

It's hard to make sense of something that seems as silly as a fear of cheeseburgers, but try to see things from your loved one's perspective if you can—it's not about the food, remember? Kristen, 25, from Wisconsin said that it's important to try to understand what your loved one is going through, as well as the events that led up to their eating disorder, in order to get an idea of everything they've been through. She added that beyond doing that, the most important thing is to simply let your loved one know you care about them.

Questions Friends & Family Should Ask

1. What kinds of foods are most challenging for you to eat? What can we do to help you feel more comfortable with them?

2. How can we plan to help you feel more comfortable eating with other people?

3. What can we do to help you feel more relaxed during the holidays, or other times when you come to visit?

Journal Questions for Friends & Family

4. What seem to be some of my loved one's specific eating challenges? How can I be supportive throughout these?

5. How can I help him or her feel more comfortable in social eating situations? What are some things I can do, and positive phrases I can say?

6. What are some holiday traditions we can start that aren't related to food? What are some fun activities we can do at other times when the family gathers?

Q & A with Barbara Truitt

Q: What advice would you give to someone just learning to eat with their loved ones again?

A: When you eat with your family, set aside your mind and focus on everyone at the table. Ask each person how their day went. Talk about TV shows, songs, or movies.

It is important to lay down some "temporary rules"—I say temporary because people with eating disorders tend to latch on to these rules too long. The rules are usually as follows (and feel free to add some of your own):

1. Please do not talk about food at this meal.

2. Please refrain from conversation using the words "skinny," "fat," and "bad."

3. Do not talk about meals previously eaten at any time.

4. Do not talk about clothes being too big or too small on anyone.

5. Do not talk about restaurants or fast food places.

6. (Pick your biggest trigger and add that to the list).

Use these rules for at least two months, and then each week, take away one rule at a time.

8 It Won't Go to Your Hips: Building a better body (image)

"Since love grows within you, so beauty grows. For love is the beauty of the soul."

–Saint Augustine

I was the ripe old age of eight when I suddenly started noticing some weird things going on with my body. I'll spare you most of the gory details, but within the span of a year, I had grown bigger than most of the kids in my grade, and was even a head taller than my year-and-a-half older brother (frustrating for *both* of us!). By middle school, thanks to the early curves I'd developed, I was already getting noticed by high school guys who assumed I was a college student. Despite that, I was secretly a little jealous of the smaller girls in my class, who looked so dainty and always seemed to get more attention from the boys my age.

When I started my first diet in high school, I had a "magic number" weight range in my head that I thought I needed to reach in order to be the perfect size. I came up with that number based on weights I had seen listed for actresses, models, and all those happy women I read about in magazine weight loss articles. I didn't think about the fact that my body probably wasn't supposed to be in that weight range, or that I shouldn't even have been paying any attention to those numbers anyway: Women are notorious for stretching the truth about their weight a little bit, so who knows how many of the weight loss articles actually had legitimate numbers in them in the first place? And as for the models and actresses I saw, it's pretty unlikely that very many of them were even at a healthy weight.

No matter how glamorous some people think it is to be skinny, it was when I was at my lowest weight that I felt the *least* beautiful. Although I was more emotionally "comfortable" being underweight, I still didn't like the shape of my thighs, or the fact that I was probably wearing the same size bra that I wore as a 6th grader. My muscles were weak, and I was too self-conscious about my bony shoulders to ever wear tank tops or strapless dresses in public.

Still, a couple of years ago when I told one of my friends I wanted to gain weight, she gave me a look that was somewhat of a cross between shock and horror: "You *what?*" she asked. She knitted her eyebrows together and thought for a moment before speaking again. "I mean…I just don't know where it would *go!*"

It's hard to strengthen your resolve when people are saying things like that to you. It also didn't help that I was a little afraid if I just let myself eat what I wanted, I might somehow transform back into the chubby, unsure girl I envisioned myself to be back in high school. After my friend said that to me, I found myself gazing down at my body for the rest of the day, trying to figure out whether she was right. Maybe I *was* being ridiculous for thinking I needed to eat more—I mean, I still had a butt, and I still didn't like my stomach all that much. And it wasn't exactly like I had lost any *more* weight over the past couple of years, even if I was "technically" underweight.

Beyond that, it seemed like I was constantly being praised for my thinness. A few months earlier, a trainer at my gym complimented me on my "lean" body, and asked me what my diet was like. I told him that I believed in everything in moderation, but in my head I was really thinking about how obsessively I tracked my calories throughout the day, and how I often threw away portions of my food before I had the chance to eat it. I thought it was ironic that he was so interested in how I got my "figure," when at the time *I* was more concerned about finding gym shirts that didn't just hang awkwardly over my scrawny ribs.

It's unfortunate that in today's society, being underweight is actually considered by many to be a mark of fitness. There are so many girls and women—and now men!—who are very thin that it's almost considered commonplace, instead of concerning. If the friend I mentioned earlier couldn't picture me at a healthier weight, it was only because she had never met me before I had an eating disorder. She didn't know that I hadn't had a real period in years, or that I felt lightheaded every time I tried to work out, or that contrary to what she'd probably always heard, thinner most definitely *isn't* better when it comes to health or happiness.

Even if you think you're at an acceptable weight, there may be things going on in your body that indicate otherwise. Here are a few things to keep in mind:

Take an Honest Look at Your Body (and Health)

First things first: **You have to be at a healthy weight** if you really want to recover. You need to be healthy if you want the energy, ability, and focus that will allow you to truly pursue your passions and live your life. Your body is your ally—not the enemy. What's a healthy weight for you? Keep reading this chapter!

Defeat denial of the seriousness of your weight issues. With all of the talk out there about extreme fitness and restrictive special diets, it can be easy to justify obsessions with your eating, gym routines, or body fat levels. This can be especially true for guys, whose disordered eating and exercise habits often go completely unrecognized. No matter how "healthy" you believe your habits are, if you wake up feeling weak and exhausted every morning, if you have trouble focusing and achieving tasks throughout the day, or if you're a female of reproductive age and not having a *real*, normal menstrual cycle, you're still not where you need to be.

I have to apologize and say that the next section is mostly geared towards women, but it illustrates some knowledge I gained that greatly impacted the way I view my own health, in terms of the way my body functions. Please also note that this is your cue to skip the next few paragraphs if you want to avoid some mild TMI!

It wasn't until I read a book called *Taking Charge of Your Fertility*, by Toni Weschler, that the truth about my body really hit home with me. I knew I was underweight, even if it wasn't extreme. I knew I wasn't having a period and that that probably wasn't the healthiest thing in the world. But for some crazy reason, even without a monthly cycle, I still thought it would be possible for me to get pregnant someday. I'd heard plenty of stories about women who never got periods being suddenly surprised by pregnancies, including a close friend of mine. So I naturally assumed that having a period wasn't a requirement for becoming a mother in the natural way.

I was wrong—well, sort of. I learned that even though it is possible for a woman who isn't menstruating regularly to sporadically ovulate, that might only happen once in a blue moon. I wasn't willing to gamble on whether or not that blue moon might actually appear for *me*. In Weschler's book, she teaches you how to chart changes in your body using the Fertility Awareness Method (FAM), so you know what's actually going on with your cycle—or what's *not* going on. It is similar to Natural Family Planning (NFP), which is taught to couples who are planning on getting married in the Roman Catholic Church. I have to admit that even though I attempted to chart a few times after my husband and I attended our own NFP classes, I had some trouble understanding some of my individual issues until I read Weschler's book.

If you are female, I highly suggest you look into FAM and NFP (Natural Family Planning resources can be found at The Couple to Couple League website, at http://www.ccli.org/).While my beliefs are more in line with NFP, it was through the information I received from sources associated with both methods that I was able to begin gaining a more comprehensive picture of what was going on with my body—or I should say, what *wasn't* going on with it, until after I started getting back to a healthy weight.

Even a brief amount of research will reveal that women often have cycle disturbances if they are experiencing emotional or physical stress. Physical stress can be in the form of exercising too much, not getting enough sleep, or not eating properly. Your cycle can be impacted even if you are not underweight: If you're not giving yourself the right balance of nutrition and rest, it won't be able to function as well.

It's important to note that even after you begin decreasing the physical stress on your body (by increasing your calories, exercising less, and/or gaining weight, depending on your individual situation), it may take some time until you are regular again. Further, if the balance of diet, exercise, and weight continues to be insufficient, your body may not be functioning in a way that will allow you to achieve or sustain a healthy pregnancy, even if your cycles seem "normal" on the surface. Finally, please remember that just as everyone's bodies are different, everyone's individual needs are different: Even though there are some general understandings of what is helpful for women in recovery, the balance of nutrition and exercise that works best for me or others might not work the same way for you. Along with your own research, please consult your own physician and dietitian when trying to figure out what *your* body needs.

I had to change my habits not only because it's what I needed to do to be healthy, but because I care very deeply about my relationship with my husband and the future we hope to have together. I care so much more about that than I do about being ridiculously thin. Reading that book was like suddenly becoming aware of the fact that there were colors in the world that I had never seen before. It completely changed the way I think about my body.

Okay, so I have to stop for a moment here and complicate things a little bit (sorry!). I really mean it when I say charting has changed the way I think about my health. I've learned things about my body that I never would have discovered if I hadn't begun doing it. However, the process isn't without challenges. I will do my best to explain: One of the three major fertility signs involved in charting is the shift in your basal body temperature that occurs immediately after ovulation. Even though you can track other things, it is the most reliable way to see whether you are actually ovulating or not (as opposed to having a non-ovulatory cycle that may closely resemble a normal cycle). It can also tell you whether or not your cycle is balanced.

Here's where it gets a little problematic: Your temperature is a number, just like calories, fat grams, exercise minutes, or your weight (the last two of which I'll talk about later on in this chapter). After charting for a few cycles, I (and my poor husband!) realized I was starting to get a little too focused on it. I started overthinking and worrying about every little fluctuation, to the point where I was having trouble concentrating on other things. That temperature I took in the morning was beginning to affect my day, just like my weight used to do when I still weighed myself. I think tracking my temperature was an amazing way for me to get a sense of what was going on in my body, but there came a point when my husband and I both decided it would be best if I took a break from the temperature-taking component for awhile. Even now, I still only track my temperature at certain points during my cycle.

If you begin charting, it's incredibly important to be aware of how it is affecting you emotionally. You can learn some remarkable things about your body throughout the process, but it's only helpful so long as you feel empowered and enlightened by it, rather than just mildly crazy (like I felt for awhile!).

But let's get back on our original path again: If you're a woman of childbearing age, don't take your fertility lightly: The longer you have an eating disorder, the more difficult it may be for you to get pregnant and/or sustain a healthy pregnancy. I sincerely urge you to start figuring out what's going on with *your* body and try to get everything back on track as soon as possible. Your chances of being a mother may depend on it.

If you're a guy, you don't automatically have a "Get out of Jail Free" card here: Your diet and lifestyle also have a major impact on your health and fertility. If you are interested, Marilyn M. Shannon's book, *Fertility, Cycles, & Nutrition* contains some great advice for you, too.

What if you *don't* want to get pregnant? Does any of this even matter at all? No matter what your aspirations are, it is still important to be aware of what's going on with your body, because your cycle can be an important indicator of your health. You won't be able to reach your peak energy or performance level until your body is balanced. Also, if you *aren't* prepared to be a mother, as I said earlier, you can still get pregnant before you have a period, because it is still possible for you to ovulate without expecting it.

Whether you're old or young, man or woman, healthy bodyweight is important for both good health and stable emotions. **The way you treat your body today will also have a significant impact on your long-term well-being.** You wouldn't deprive a plant of water or sunlight and expect it to flourish, would you? The same goes for your body: The more you take care of yourself now, the greater your chances are of staying healthy later on in life.

Taking care of yourself comes a little more naturally once you learn to start loving the body you've been blessed with. The following section is your roadmap to better body image:

Love Your Sexy Bod

Don't obsess over certain parts of your body. Just like some of the difficulties you may have in your life, the problem areas you perceive your body to have will only seem magnified if you dwell on them. One of the biggest things that kept me from getting back to a healthy weight early on in my recovery was the fact that I was constantly "checking" certain parts of my body in the mirror to make sure they hadn't somehow spontaneously morphed into something horrible since I'd eaten or since I'd worked out last. All this constant checking made it impossible for me to just learn to listen to my body about what I should be eating and how I should be exercising. If I didn't like the way a certain part of my body looked (and I usually didn't), I would end up restricting, over-exercising, or just plain feeling bad about myself.

Keep in mind that **your view of yourself may be distorted.** It wasn't until after I got back to a healthy weight that I was really able to see how unhappy and lifeless I looked when I was at my lowest weight. I feel so much better about myself now than I ever did then—and I've heard the same thing time and time again from others who have recovered.

Remember that you are your harshest critic. Usually the people around you aren't noticing any of the "flaws" you see in your body. If they are noticing something, it might be time to make some new friends, because they're probably not the kind of people you want to be spending your time with anyway. Shannon, 22, from Texas said, "I started paying attention to others in the room. I used to think that when people were looking at me, it meant they thought I looked fat; but if I looked closely, I saw that many of them had admiring looks."

Do an emotional self-check when you start to criticize yourself. Jan Lockert, 53, from Ohio, said it wasn't until she reached a healthy weight that she was able to get a more realistic perspective of herself:

> *"Once I had restored my weight to a healthy level for my body, my perceptions and cognitive abilities quickly began to normalize. I now know that if I have a moment of discomfort that feels like it is connected to my weight or body size, I am not allowing myself to feel or express some emotion adequately. I now am able to distinctly separate my emotions from eating, weight, and body shape or size. I am confident in who I am, not based on what I weigh. That's the difference."*

Focus on developing a healthier perspective. No matter how much you weigh, you're always going to have the same body, with the same shape. Even when I was at my lowest weight, I was self-conscious about some of the proportions of my body. The best thing I've been able to do for myself has been to upcycle my perspective by focusing on what I *do* like about my body, as well as all of the wonderful things my healthy body allows me to do.

Julia Leonard, 23, from Worcestershire, England began to see the process of gaining weight as a reassurance, rather than something to be feared:

> *"Restoring your bodyweight means restoring the chemical balances in your brain, and in turn, the ability to rationalize and develop a healthy attitude toward weight gain, which becomes easier and more natural. I've learned that I cannot function at my best and reach my potential as 'Julia' below a certain BMI. It's no fun looking like half a person—you can only function as half a person! Life is much more enjoyable when you have a body to dress up and learn to be proud of."*

I've had a remarkable change in the way I think about my body, and about beauty in general. I'm not superficial like I once was, looking at all those "perfect" images of magazine models. I don't think of beauty in terms of how well it fits the mold of what I see on TV anymore. It probably won't surprise you that I think some of the most beautiful bodies in the world are the bodies of mothers: Is there anything more beautiful and amazing than the sacrifice of carrying and giving birth to a child? I know women who are very self-conscious about some of the changes their bodies went through during pregnancy, when in reality those changes are the mark of a miracle having occurred. I pray every day that I will someday be blessed to wear that badge, too.

It's not just mothers who are beautiful, but anyone who uses their bodies to live a beautiful life: The elderly man whose hands are calloused from a lifetime of helping others, the cashier at the grocery store who greets every single person she meets with a genuine smile no matter how exhausted she is, and the bright-eyed, curious toddler who saunters down the aisles of church on Sunday and lifts everyone's day.

How could anyone say that any of those people aren't beautiful? My goal is to use my body to do meaningful things every day, instead of stifling my own abilities with words and thoughts of self-hatred. **Say no to the negative thoughts that pop into your head throughout the day:** As I said in Chapter Four, one of the best things I've learned to do when I start to think something negative has been to upcycle that thought into something more positive. As soon as the words "I look fat" pop into my head, I immediately change it to "I look and *feel* good at a healthy weight," or "My body can do some amazing things."

I'm my body's friend now: The last time I found myself beginning to criticize my body (after I'd tried unsuccessfully to put on a pair of my old jeans), I immediately and without even really thinking about it, noticed myself saying to that negative voice, "Shut up! I wanted to gain weight. I look good with curves, and I feel strong. Thank God I'm healthy now." And you know what? I really mean it when I say those things now. After years of hating myself, it's a pretty incredible feeling.

Don't compare yourself to anyone but yourself. No matter how much my weight has changed throughout my life so far, one thing has stayed the same: My body. No matter how much I've exercised or how focused I've been on my diet, my natural shape hasn't changed. I feel healthier and happier when I'm getting a healthy amount of exercise and eating well, but I'll never look like anyone other than myself.

Change your perspective when you see people who are very thin. You know how women who want to have a baby always say they see pregnant women everywhere they go? When I was trying to gain weight, I felt like I saw skinny people everywhere. Sometimes I'd start to question what I was doing: Did I really need to gain weight when "everyone else" was so thin? Why was it "okay" for them to be thin, and not me?

Keep in mind that many of the very thin people you see aren't necessarily healthy—some may be, because it's impossible to know what anyone's individual circumstances are unless you know them very well (and often, not even then). However, you probably know that unhealthy eating habits are incredibly common in our society. That skinny person you just saw may be perfectly healthy, but they might also be weak and miserable. They may be struggling with an illness or some unhealthy behaviors of their own. Seeing very thin people is not a justification for you to be unhealthy.

Find healthy examples of people with positive body images. While still taking into account the fact that your body will never be the same as anyone else's, it can be helpful for you to be on the lookout for people who seem to be in a healthy weight range, and appear to be confident in themselves. Take it a step further and **make an inspirational collage:** Cut out and collect pictures of healthy, fit, happy people who represent how you want to feel as a result of your recovery. Make sure you include plenty of pictures of people who have body types that are not the kind you usually find in fashion magazines, but who still can be considered beautiful. Look at your collage when you're not feeling so body-confident, and need a little encouragement.

Another collage idea: Find some photos of yourself that you like, from a time when you were happy and doing something you love. Also include magazine or newspaper clippings with images or phrases that represent the future you hope to have, including things you love, things you want to do, places you want to go, goals you want to achieve, etc.

If you'd like, **create your own motivational magazine, to replace some of the fashion or fitness magazines that trigger you:** Fill a binder with any clippings you find that have truly healthy focuses, like recovery stories, stories that promote healthy eating rather than weight loss, or fitness articles that encourage health and fitness rather than weight loss.

Try out a new lens. The next time you're in a public place, spend some time looking for people who aren't the Hollywood "standard" of attractiveness: What kinds of special characteristics make them who they are? Do they have a unique sense of style, genuineness in their eyes, or a kind way of treating others? Focus on seeing the *people*, rather than their bodies. What kinds of characteristics do you have that you're proud of?

What are some positive features you already have that you would like to develop?

Strive to be a healthy example for others. Be proud of being healthy, so you can share that perspective with those around you, like your children, siblings, nieces and nephews, and any other young (or older!) people you may encounter. Whether you recognize it or not, they're paying attention to how you treat and talk about your body.

Develop a sense of gratitude for your body and everything it allows you to do. Amy Pettengill, 27, from New Hampshire said that although she hated how she looked and acted while she had her eating disorder, it was once she developed gratitude for her body that her whole attitude transformed:

> *"I don't wake up every morning hating myself and my body anymore. I don't feel like a failure for not spending the day obsessing. I don't 'feel fat' every day. I wake up in the morning and am grateful for the body I have, and the functions it can perform. It took several years for me to develop this gratitude. The important thing is once the gratitude came, self-acceptance followed."*

Be your body's "pen pal." Take some time to write a letter to your body: Tell your body specifically how you're going to be more accepting of and loving towards it, especially throughout some of the most difficult times in your recovery. What kinds of things are you going to do to take care of your body? What are you thankful for that your body can do? **Every day, pick out three parts of your body that you appreciate.** What do you appreciate about them? Remember to thank your body!

Turn toward your faith. Heather, 18, from New Hampshire remembers a day when she received several compliments on her beauty from total strangers. She took it as a sign that God was taking care of her throughout all her challenges:

> *"I was not becoming fat or ugly but I was becoming beautiful, inside and out, through God's saving and merciful grace. I did not think I deserved to get second chances with a body that I had spent years destroying, but God had many different and better plans for me…I really try to search for the wonderful things that God sees in me. God judges us from the inside, but we need to keep our bodies healthy in order to carry out the plans that He has for us. Instead of focusing solely on the reflection in the mirror, I focus on what the reflection in the mirror can do. I focus on the upbeat and happy personality that is beginning to shine through, and the energy that keeps me moving forward."*

Your body is not representative of who *you* are. However, it is your responsibility to keep your body as healthy as possible, so that you can use it in countless wonderful ways.

Remember that your healthy weight is different from anyone else's. If you're familiar with the Body Mass Index (BMI) scale, you may know that a healthy weight is considered anything between an 18.5 and 24.9. However, this doesn't mean you're automatically healthy if you're between those ranges. Despite initially having a goal of reaching an 18.5 BMI myself, I realized I wasn't finished when I got there, because my body was still not functioning like it needed to. **Don't rely on numbers;** your physician is the best person to tell you whether or not you're healthy (also see the next section for more thoughts on weighing yourself).

Banish your fears of becoming overweight. As long as you keep practicing those healthy eating habits, **your body will naturally find its healthy "set point."** For a few years, post-bulimia, I found myself in a bit of a trap when it came to thinking about my body and how I was eating. I hated feeling so obsessive about my diet, and it made me a little nervous that I was losing more weight than was good for me. But even more than that, I was afraid that if I really began just eating whenever my body told me to, I would inevitably get out of control and end up in the whole binge-purge cycle again. It was hard for me to really believe that as long as I simply nourished my body the right way, all those crazy food cravings would actually improve enough to where I *wasn't* thinking about food literally all day long.

For a long time, even though I had heard plenty about the whole idea of my body having a set point, I still wanted to maintain that false sense of control that came with my eating disorder. I still wanted to try to stay just a little bit underweight, because in my mind, it was "safer" to be that way. I believed that as long as I was underweight, I was protecting myself from ever having to worry about being *over*weight (that whole black-and-white way of thinking that comes with eating disorders again!). I didn't trust myself or my body to maintain that healthy balance, and so my obsession with food and my body hung on.

Thankfully, as I continued to learn more about normal eating habits over time, I learned how unrealistic all my old feelings about eating and weight actually were: Obese people don't become obese from just eating a cookie every once in awhile (or even every day), or occasionally eating a bigger meal. Even though my husband eats what I think is an insane amount sometimes, he is still able to stay at his healthy weight because he balances it out at other times, when he isn't so hungry. As long as I continue to trust my body, I will stay at my healthy weight, too. Gaining more than *your* healthy weight happens only when you overeat *consistently*—not when you're staying balanced by staying mindful of your body and its needs.

Author, parent, and advocate Doris Smeltzer pointed out to me that it's important for those who are learning to eat intuitively to remember that there are natural variations of healthy bodyweight:

> *"Becoming 'overweight' may have nothing to do with 'overeating.' Some people have a large body due to the genes they inherited—they may eat 'normally' and be metabolically-fit, yet 'overweight.' Some medications cause weight gain, and sometimes socioeconomic status determines the quality and amount of food available. We come in diverse sizes for many reasons. The important thing is to know that we can strive toward health no matter what body size we may have."*

Need more convincing that health comes in different sizes? On page 108 of the book I mentioned earlier, Shannon's *Fertility, Cycles, & Nutrition*, she describes how "seemingly sensible weight loss" negatively impacted (or stopped) the menstrual cycles of otherwise healthy women. Why? Despite maintaining supposedly "ideal" weights, their bodies were actually below their individual *natural* healthy weight ranges. Shannon says their cycles normalized after they regained a few pounds. In a society so obsessed with being thin, this is a concept that can be hard to wrap your mind around! However, it illustrates the fact that you really can't look at your health in terms of how well you fit into a specific weight range, BMI category, or jean size: Your body knows where it needs to be, more than any online calculator or table in the back of a book.

You'll find more thoughts from contributors about their healthy weights later on in this chapter. You'll also find their thoughts on why the scale really is so detrimental to recovery.

Don't get discouraged if you think you've gained too much weight, or that you've gained weight too quickly. As long as you stick to your meal plan and keep working on recognizing and responding to your body's hunger signals, everything will even out. It just takes time.

Lindsey Wert, 24, from California, said that her body's healthy changes came with a whole new perspective on life:

> *"I have seen how resilient the mind and body can be, after nearly a decade of torture and malnutrition. The body is miraculous. It knows what it needs, what it needs to weigh, and how to heal when it's hurt. The body is the smartest thing there is. As I begin to take care of my body, mind, heart, and soul, I am able to experience sensation, touch, and movement in a capacity that never existed before. My intuition is my soul's guide. I did not know of this existence before recovery."*

Feeling more comfortable in your own skin is a gradual process; until then, make it a point to **dress comfortably.** Wear clothes that let you move and breathe, and don't keep anything that doesn't fit you anymore. It's almost impossible to feel comfortable if you're still trying to tug on a pair of jeans you wore when you were at an unhealthy size. For me this usually meant dropping off my old jeans at a thrift store, or even pulling out the scissors and slicing them all up and down the sides before I could change my mind and try to wear them again. My husband was also wonderful about reminding me that I didn't *need* to fit into a pair of jeans that probably belonged in the closet of someone half my age!

Dress well—even (and especially!) if it's only for yourself. Put on clothes that make you feel good about yourself every day, even if you're just going to stay at home alone.

Nicole Geddie, 24, from New Mexico said it helped her a great deal to **come up with two "safe" outfits:**

> *"I have a very hard time just getting dressed in the morning, because everything I put on tends to make me feel bad about myself. I have two outfits that have saved me on days when I'm ready to give up and crawl in a corner and cry myself to death. It's really important to have a safety net available for yourself in times when hopelessness creeps in (and it WILL happen, no matter how far along in recovery you may be!)."*

Amy Pettengill, 27, from New Hampshire said she found a brand of jeans she always felt comfortable in, and then bought seven pairs in seven different shades.

Jennifer, 30, from Missouri learned to **shop at Goodwill for clothes.** She added that it's also a lot easier to get rid of clothes when you haven't spent a lot of money on them:

> *"Not only does it save you money, but it really helped me to realize how crazy sizes are in different brands. For example, I can go to Goodwill, pick out 10 pairs of jeans to try on in many different sizes, and find that sizes really do vary. This helped me to really realize that I'm not defined by numbers…When I got to a weight that my therapist and I agreed was healthy, I cleaned out my closet and gave all my 'thin clothes' to the Hurricane Katrina victims. That was a defining moment for me, and it also helped me move forward."*

No matter where you choose to shop, **stop looking at clothing size labels,** like Andrea Roe, 28, from British Columbia, Canada did:

> *"I was very obsessed with the clothing size I could fit or squeeze myself into. Something that helped me overcome this was to cut out all the labels of my clothes. And whenever I went clothes shopping with my mum (who of course knew about my eating disorder and body image issues), I'd go in the changing room and she'd bring me clothes to try on so I never looked at the size labels. I had no idea what sizes I was trying on, and that was very liberating. As soon as we arrived at home, she'd cut out all the labels before I put the clothes away in my cupboard. It's something very simple, but helped me a lot to take my mind off of the 'size obsession.'"*

Only buy clothes that you know you love. This is probably one of the biggest things for me: Much of the reason I didn't feel good about myself when I was younger was probably because I always shopped in a hurry, without really trying things on, and I focused too much on buying cheap clothes over those that looked nice on me. I'd buy five cheap, ugly, and ill-fitting pairs of jeans instead of one or two really nice pairs. This was a complete losing situation for me: Not only did most of what I took home look less-than-wonderful on me, but a lot of it just ended up hanging unworn in my closet. Now, I'm much more about quality than quantity. I have a rule that I don't buy anything unless I'm 100% sure I love it. That's not saying I just buy expensive clothes all the time, because I still hate spending extra money if I don't have to. Most of the things I buy are on sale, but their prices aren't the main indicator of whether or not I buy them anymore. I make sure I try everything on, and if it doesn't look good on me, it's not worth the money—even if it is only a couple of dollars.

Find your own style instead of trying to look like everyone else. Enjoy yourself and go shopping for clothes in fun colors, and that accent your favorite parts. For the ladies, find some colorful makeup that shows off your eyes, and glittery nail polish that will complete your look and make you feel put together. Guys can find unique shoes or all kinds of fun ties, with all sorts of crazy colors, images, and patterns.

Try something new! Rachelle, 23, from Arizona said there was a day in treatment when they had to talk about one thing related to their physical appearance that they would never let themselves do or be seen doing, and then challenge those ideas:

> *"I said I would never let my hair go curly, since I hated it. We then had to come the next day doing whatever we had said, just to see that there is nothing wrong with it. I found that I actually liked my hair that way, and got compliments on it. It made me realize that I need to try new things, and try things that I was once afraid of, because I won't know the result until I do."*

Is there something you've always said you would never wear, or never do with your hair? Why not give it a shot and see what happens?

Set yourself up for success. Don't read magazines with advertisements that make you feel bad about yourself, or articles about weight loss. Surround yourself with people who are good for your body image and don't constantly talk about calories and dieting.

Wear confidence—the sexiest accessory. When you feel good about the way you look, other people will see it too. If you want an instant makeover, try simply smiling. That, combined with wearing clothes that make you feel good, makes you instantly attractive. **Thank people for their compliments** instead of brushing them off, and write down what they've said in a journal or on sticky notes that you can post up all over your room to remember on a bad day. **Recognize others for their**

positive features, abilities, and actions; after all, one of the best ways to get a compliment is to give one!

Be mindful of how your emotions affect your body image. I've noticed that some of the times I start to feel "fat" are when there's a lot going on around me and I'm feeling overwhelmed. I start to crave control over my body when I don't feel like I can control anything else in my life. The key for me is to take note of what's going on in my emotional life, so I can make a plan for how to respond to it in a healthy way.

Also remember that if you do feel a little insecure about how you look sometimes, it's important to talk honestly about it with the people you love. **Don't try to get reactions from others by asking those loaded questions,** like "Do you think I look like I've gained weight?", or making disparaging comments about your body. Even though other people can be very supportive, ultimately, it's your job to make yourself feel good about how you look and who you are—not theirs.

Resist the urge to weigh yourself. Why? Keep on reading…

Rethink Your Weight

I probably started weighing myself in 6th grade, when my brother and I first discovered an old dial scale in my grandma's bedroom. It was fun for us to see how much we weighed when we went to visit her. At that time, it was more of a novelty than anything. Even in middle school when I felt kind of chubby, the number didn't really bother me that much.

I still remember the day my parents bought a couple of scales for our house—one for their bathroom, and one for my brother's and mine. They were slim white digital scales we had picked up after a day of shopping. I had had a big strawberry milkshake on the drive home. Just moments after we parked our car in the garage, my brother and I had removed our scale from its packaging and placed it down on our bathroom floor to try it out. I was quite surprised by the number I saw. When I saw it, I remember thinking about all the other numbers my friends at school were constantly talking about, and all the numbers I saw in fitness magazines—numbers that were definitely lower than mine.

That was the night I began my first diet. Two years later, after numerous failed diets and exercise plans, I stepped over the threshold into bulimia.

As you probably already know, the only thing bulimia does is make your weight go crazy. There's no way for you to know how much your body is actually absorbing, and because your body doesn't know how to respond to what you're doing to it, your metabolism gets all out of whack. When I finally stopped bingeing and purging, my metabolism was so poor that it only reinforced my belief that my body was just "different" from everybody else's somehow. It seemed like I gained weight any time I ever ate more than just a little bit.

As I've said at other points in this book, it wasn't long into my recovery from bulimia that I began slowly sliding in the other direction, towards anorexia. At that time, my compulsion to weigh myself grew from just doing it in the morning, to doing it several times throughout the day. Some days, as I looked at how low the number dipped, I'd get a little lightheaded and my heart would begin to pound—but despite my fears about how much my body was wasting away, I was somehow even more afraid to just eat normally. I used the scale to tell me how much to eat, instead of listening to my body.

It's no surprise that all that weighing had such a negative effect on me; after all, **numbers feed disordered thoughts.** When you have numbers like weights, calories, and exercise minutes constantly floating around in your head, it all acts like a giant smokescreen so you can't hear what your body is trying to tell you.

Your weight shouldn't impact how you feel about yourself. Ashley Devitt, 18, from Florida remembers a nurse she had in treatment who said to her, "Why do you give the scale so much power and let it determine your self-worth? Imagine if I told you my self-worth was determined by the toaster. Sound crazy, huh?" Ashley said the nurse proved her point, and that after that she got rid of all of the scales in her house to help her avoid temptation.

Weighing is just another unhealthy coping mechanism. You may feel more compelled to step on the scale if you're frustrated, sad, or anxious, even if you know that doing so may very well make you feel even worse. See Chapter Four for some healthier ways to deal with tough emotions.

Your weight is not a reliable number. All kinds of things will cause it to fluctuate. Brittany, 26, from Maryland said, "It took me years to realize your body fluctuates in the amount you weigh even if you eat the same thing every day for a month! It is important to remember that salt intake, water intake, and your menstrual cycle can greatly affect the amount that you weigh from day to day."

Your weight can affect more than your mood. On days when you've seen a higher weight than you wanted on your scale, how has that impacted the rest of your day? How has it affected how you chose to spend your time and the way you interacted with other people?

Here's how you can free yourself from the scale, and still stay fit:

Banish the Scale

Listen to and trust your body. Your body really isn't that different from everyone else's. The only reason I ever gained weight throughout my years of on and off dieting was because I wasn't practicing healthy eating habits; I would starve myself some days, and then eat everything in sight on others. And the only reason I temporarily gained weight after I stopped bingeing and purging was because my digestive system hadn't yet recovered from all of the damage I'd done to it. **Your metabolism will improve as long as you keep eating healthily.** Once I began finally allowing myself to just eat a nutritious, balanced diet, I was surprised by how much I could actually eat without gaining weight. Now, as long as I'm paying attention to my body and its hunger signals, I know just what to eat and how much to exercise to keep myself fit and happy.

Not sure how to start? **Your meal plan will teach you how to eat**, even if you haven't eaten normally in years (Check out Chapter Six if you haven't already).

Have fun getting rid of your scale. Give it a ceremonial burial in your backyard, or smash it with a hammer before you throw it away. **Give it to someone else to throw away for you** if you don't think you will follow through with it on your own.

Redecorate your bathroom like Hilary, 27, from California did. According to her, "…there were so many negative memories associated with that space. I needed to erase that negativity that was associated with that part of the house." Ellen, 26, from New York suggested putting a picture of a scale where yours used to be and writing something inspirational on it, like, "A scale cannot measure my worth."

Trust your physician to help you make sure you stay at a healthy weight, but **stand with your back to the scale when you visit the doctor's office.** I know this is easier said than done, especially if you sometimes feel like your weight is the only thing you have any "control" over in your life. As tough as it may be at first, it's an essential step in recovery, because that number is actually controlling *you.* Trust your medical team; it's their job to keep you as healthy as possible.

Find better ways to gauge your fitness, like paying attention to how you're feeling on a daily basis and going for regular checkups with your physician. Keep track of how your workouts are progressing and what your energy level is like throughout the day. As long as you stay mindful and keep responding to your physical and emotional feelings in a healthy way, you'll be able to keep yourself as healthy as possible, and your physician will help you make sure of it.

Also**, be smart about working out.** Contrary to what you may have heard in the media, exercise actually doesn't have to feel a little like self-torture for you in order for you to reap the benefits. Here's how you can make exercise your friend while in recovery:

Exercise Wisely

Despite all the health benefits associated with regular exercise, you have to **wait until you're healthy** to do it. Make sure you are at *your* healthy weight, and get your doctor's permission first. Exercising before your body is ready will only cause further damage to your body. Remember that even after you have your physician's approval to begin exercising, you may have to **set limits on your workouts.** Especially after having experienced an eating disorder, **you may overestimate the amount of physical activity that is healthy for your body.** Because your body is in a state of repair, you may be able to tolerate less physical exertion than other people. Feeling excessively tired, moody, or unable to concentrate throughout the day may be signs that your body is not getting the rest that it needs. Along with the proper nutrition, be sure to **balance your exercise with plenty of sleep.** This will help your body be able to recover more quickly from your workouts.

Troy Roness, 23, from North Dakota, acknowledged that it can be difficult for anyone, and especially males, to be able to distinguish good and bad fitness and eating habits:

> *"There's such a huge push for the perfect body; to become that lean, fit and muscular individual, that the majority of sufferers don't think of their habits as unhealthy. A few things that I have learned over time are that if you are exercising for any reason other than for enjoyment, changing your eating patterns (even slightly) to fit in, or pushing yourself in a direction for approval from someone else; those are huge red flags."*

Be honest about your habits if you have the tendency to over-exercise, and visit with your counselor about alternative things you can do to relax and relieve anxiety and other tough emotions (how about using that "Alternative Activity" list I keep mentioning from Chapter One?).

Exercise with a friend or family member, as long as you both agree on what a healthy and appropriate amount of exercise is; this will not only help you enjoy your workout more, but it will also keep you accountable. **Stick to your workout limits by scheduling specific fitness classes in your planner or going to the gym only when you have a set period of time**, like on your lunch break or before work. Nicole Geddie, 24, from New Mexico said she keeps her tendency to over-exercise in check by scheduling in other activities right after her workouts:

> *"I tend to push myself past my limits, especially if I am working out with someone or at a gym around other athletes, because I automatically think that I should be keeping up with the marathon runners. Something that works for me, is to schedule something (coffee with a friend, etc.), and do my workout right beforehand, so that I absolutely have to stop exercising at a certain time no matter what."*

Only allow yourself to exercise if you've met your other recovery

goals, like following your meal plan without resorting to any old disordered behaviors. Instead of sticking to a rigid routine, **try some new types of exercise,** and think about having fun and being healthy instead of burning calories. How about a partner dance class, yoga, or tai chi?

Be realistic about the effect that exercise has on your body. Again, even though a moderate amount is wonderful and healthy, it in itself isn't going to give you a different body. **Listen to your body's signals** so you can recognize if you are working out too much, and **don't be afraid to take some time off from working out for awhile.** I used to never go a day without exercising, no matter how tired and weak I felt. Even though I always spaced my weightlifting workouts to try to give my muscles some time to recover, I still always did some sort of workout. When I lifted weights I did the same specific exercises every single week, even though I got so sick of them that I literally began to dread doing them. I thought I'd get out of shape if I didn't do those same exercises. When I finally came to my senses and realized I needed to take a break, I was amazed to find that not only did my body *not* turn into a giant marshmallow, but it actually looked better from getting the rest and recovery time it needed!

Now, even though lifting weights is still my preferred way to keep my body strong and fit, I try to include other kinds of exercise so I stay balanced and don't get into a boring rut. Sometimes my exercise is something as simple as hula hooping (I love it!) or even shopping for the day with my husband or a friend. I have a rule for myself that I don't ever do my normal workout routine if I'm feeling overly tired or really dreading it beforehand. Usually that's my body telling me to take a break. I might go for a walk or do some other kind of light activity just to energize myself, but I don't force myself to do anything I don't feel like doing.

Then, when I do choose to go back to the gym, it actually feels more like a "playground" to me again. My workouts have become my regular way to feel like I'm at recess for the day, instead of stuck in some sort of ritualistic torture!

I'm a lot happier since I stopped always saying no to doing fun things with family and friends, just because of some rigid workout schedule. If you feel like you're stuck in a bit of a rut, there are tons of fun, meaningful things you can do to get out of it—check out Chapter Three for some ideas!

Suzanne Yerdon Lewandowski, 55, from Massachusetts shared how her daily exercise transformed in recovery:

> *"...my senses became alive once the eating disorder was no longer in control. I began walking every morning—not running, just a brisk walk around the neighborhood before work. Instead of counting calories in my mind, I began looking at each house, each yard and taking in the details. I tried to imagine the insides of the homes and whether I would like living there. Varying the routes prevented*

monotony and I learned more about each neighborhood. As the seasons changed, I surmised about the family's personalities by the way they cared for their property. I waved to people, learned their habits, occasionally chatted, and made new friends. Time was not just passing me by as I worked to remain fit.

"I felt the warmth of a summer's dawn, cherished the chill of a golden autumn morning, enjoyed the crunch of snow under my boots as my parka actually kept me warm. When the world awakened in spring, I could appreciate nature's simple changes on a daily basis, breathe in the fragrance of hyacinths and lilacs, and hear the song birds return. As recovery progressed and ambitions ventured, problems and solutions were contemplated as I walked. When angry, I recall walking more purposefully; when content, the strides were slower and easier. I always felt good when done."

You miss out on a lot of life when you're too focused on your body to experience everything else that's out there. Now that I'm working with my body instead of against it, life also *feels* different. I feel at peace more than I ever have before. I am freer and able to experience life. I can linger in conversation after dinner, instead of trying to figure out where I'm going to fit in an extra workout to "make up" for the pastry I ate that I hadn't included in my plan for the day. An extra goodie here and there isn't going to get me off track, and **I know that I'll always find time for the right amount of exercise, because it's part of taking care of my body.** Not exercising isn't being any nicer to your body than over-exercising. I'm happiest and most energetic when I'm keeping that balance.

Celebrate the beauty of your recovered body. Amy Watson, 35, from Connecticut, said people noticed a new glow in her once she recovered:

"I feel and look 10 years younger now—my skin, my hair, and my nails all are so much healthier; I remember a friend telling me how radiant I look and that to me is the best compliment anyone can ever receive. No one had ever told me that before and I hold onto that compliment as motivation sometimes!"

Ali, 18, from Vermont noticed she had more energy during the day and that she felt stronger during track competitions:

"I had been worried that putting on weight would make me slower, fatter, and lazy; however, I actually ran my fastest race ever that year, because my body had sufficient fuel to build muscle and recover after exercise. The extra weight wasn't just 'fat'—it was muscle, and it was necessary for me to have the energy to train and just exist. I also felt stronger, and I wasn't pushed around as easily while playing basketball."

My whole life has turned around since I got my healthy body back. I can write and think better, and I actually have energy to chase my nephews around the house and play basketball with my husband. I still can't believe I spent so many days being unable to do that at all. Life is sad and lame when you're skinny and exhausted. Not to mention the fact that I love having curves and wearing cute, girly clothes again—Yay for being healthy!

So where do you go from here? After all these pages of tips and thoughts from so many people, what's the bottom line to achieving a truly healthy, fulfilling life?

Strike that Balance

One of my favorite ideas about health and body image was introduced to me in the book *Weightless,* by Kate Wicker, a faith-based, Catholic perspective on eating disorder recovery. In one of her final chapters, Wicker talks about the idea of temperance as a virtue. Temperance basically means acting with balance in all areas of your life—whether that be the food you eat, the exercise you do, how much you sleep or work, or anything else. Food, exercise, sleep, and work are all very wonderful things, but if one of them begins to have too much importance in your life, other areas will suffer. A balanced life is a peaceful, satisfied life—and a balanced life creates a healthy, balanced body.

Now that I'm at a healthy weight I not only feel better physically, but I actually like my body a whole lot more. Yes, there are moments when I feel puffy and gross (who doesn't have those?), but overall my muscles have more shape, I look better in all of my clothes, and I have the energy and desire to actually *do* things. I love my curves and I can wear clothes I was afraid to wear before.

My body is just another wonderful part of who I am. Even if I sometimes start to wish I had scrawnier thighs, I know they are mine and my husband loves them (he actually loves my whole body so much more now that I'm not underweight anymore!). No matter what number I might see if I stepped on a scale, I know my body is strong and beautiful and healthy. And as much as I could worry about any little wrinkle that might be starting to kiss my skin, I know that each of those little contours is just a tribute to all of the life I've lived—every laugh I've had, every vivid expression, every deep thought.

When I start looking critically at my body, I remind myself of what's really important to me. I don't want to be calculating calories over and over in my head while I'm holding my precious nephews, and completely missing the way their little faces light up with gigantic smiles as they gaze up at me. I don't want to be so focused on beating my body into shape at the gym that I wouldn't notice if someone I passed on the way needed to talk about something. For me personally, it's when I begin to criticize my body that I know I need to take a moment, reflect on my life and what's really important to me, and open up my heart to God and to those around me.

I can't help anyone when I'm hurting myself. Those in life who really matter will always see beauty when they look at me, both because of who I am inside and because I carry myself in a way that shows I am truly proud of my own individual look. My goal is to stay as healthy as possible, not only as a gift to myself, but also so I can live a long and active life with those I love.

Here are your final journal questions, followed by some additional family tips and one last Q & A section:

Journal Questions

1. What are some parts of my body I have difficulty finding beauty in? How can I begin to look at these parts of my body in a more positive way?

2. Who are some people in my life or in the media with truly healthy bodies I can look up to? How are they able to convey confidence in their more natural appearances? How can I aspire to be more like them?

3. How did I naturally move as a child? What physical activities did I enjoy? Which of those activities can I do now, in moderation?

4. What was life like before I started obsessing about my weight? Or, what *could* my life be like once I'm not spending all my time thinking about my weight?

5. What are some things I can do to reduce my temptation to weigh myself (For example, giving my scale away, asking family members to put their scales where I won't see them, or asking my doctor to weigh me backwards and not tell me the number)?

Tips for Friends & Family

Be a positive example.

Remember that your habits can be a positive influence: It was easier for me to start being more loving towards my own body once my family started talking more positively about themselves and body image in general. Once my parents began eating healthier and not keeping so much junk food around the house, it was easier for me to go home and visit without feeling triggered. We also began taking walks and doing other fun things outside together, instead of me just going somewhere and exercising by myself.

Don't bite on "Loaded Questions."

Beware of any questions (or even "casual" comments) related to weight, dieting, exercise, or anything else related to your loved one's disorder. It's not your job to constantly reassure them that their thighs don't look "fat" if they're always complaining about them. Even though it's nice if you can help them feel better about their bodies, ultimately, it's up to them to actually accept the way they look. If they ask you what weight range you think they "should" be in, just remind them that as long as they're eating in a healthy and balanced way, they won't ever have to worry about weight.

Focus on health instead of weight.

Remind your loved one how good it will feel to have energy to play the sport they love, to be able to think clearly and work productively, or to be healthy enough to raise a happy family. Don't try to encourage them by telling them how much better they'd look at a healthier weight: Even though it is important for them to reach their own *individual* ideal weight, it's usually more helpful to their recoveries if they're trying to make changes for reasons that go well beyond their appearance.

Questions Friends & Family Should Ask

1. What do you think is beautiful about you?

2. Who are some healthy people you look up to?

3. What are some things your body can do that you appreciate?

Journal Questions for Friends & Family

1. How can I respond if my loved one asks me a question about how they look? What if they make a negative comment about their weight?

2. How is my body image? How can I set a healthy example?

3. How can I adopt (or maintain) healthy exercise habits in my own life?

Q & A with Carolyn Costin, MFT, M.ED, and Keesha Broome, M.A., MFT

Q: What advice do you have for those who feel compelled to frequently weigh themselves?

A: We believe in complete abstinence from the scale. Scales have become modern-day torture devices for the women and men who use them constantly and consistently. At our treatment centers, we encourage people to let go of weighing themselves altogether, leaving this up to their treatment team to monitor. Even when going to the doctor, we advocate for getting a blind weight. The reason for our staunch belief in giving up the scale is that when someone gets into the habit of weighing himself or herself, he or she often becomes fixated on that number—Is it too high? Is it low enough? How has it changed from yesterday or this morning?

Scale weight changes from day to day; therefore, it can give false impressions...it might show that you are a pound or two up when it is really just the type of food digesting more slowly, or that you've had more sodium, or are wearing different clothes, or using a different scale. People can become slaves to this number. There can be a direct link between the number on the scale and the frequency or intensity of eating disorder behaviors. Ask yourself what you will do with the information you're given from the scale and go through the different scenarios in your head. There is never a reason good enough to weigh yourself.

Our clients repeatedly tell us that letting go of weighing was a key to their recovery. We want to free people of this obsession and suggest finding someone to help you wean yourself off of the scale. We want to encourage them to break their ties to the scale. We want people to know that the size of their heart, the worth of their soul, and the value that they have, cannot be measured by a number on a scale.

Q: What are your thoughts on physical activity during recovery?

A: Exercise is frequently tied to someone's eating disorder, but there is no possible way to give general guidelines. People in recovery may be in various physical conditions; therefore, for each person there might be a different regimen. Plus, people often like different things. We believe you need help figuring out what works best for you. And this often means being monitored and discussed with a treatment team. At times, activity might need to be seriously limited. Then as you are eating better and getting healthier and stronger, you can add exercise.

We also encourage our clients to reframe what it means to be active. Rather than running on a treadmill, take your dog on a walk. Rather than sweating through an aerobics class, play miniature golf with your family. Rather than lifting weights in a gym, take your partner bowling. There are many ways to lead an active life without sacrificing or jeopardizing your recovery. For someone who doesn't feel capable of making these swaps and wants to hold on to traditional exercise, it can be helpful to come up with an exercise contract. At our treatment centers, we believe in incorporating exercise in a balanced, moderate way and *encourage* our clients to commit to this moderation upon discharge. The regimen we shoot for at Monte Nido is three 30-minute walks per week, light weight training, and yoga. Later, if appropriate, people vary this, add to it, etc. Again, we feel it is helpful to have a professional overseeing this.

Bringing it all Together

There's a snow globe sitting on my nightstand. I keep it there year-round, even when it's a hundred degrees outside. My husband raised an eyebrow at me when we were packing up all of our things to move across the country together, because I had refused to put it in the box of holiday decorations we were planning on leaving in storage with our families.

I got the snow globe at a Christmas store in Wyoming a few years ago, when my family and I were visiting relatives. Everyone knew how crazy I am about Christmas, so we made a special trip just to go there. As we walked through the front door, my aunt and cousin told my sister and me to look around and pick out anything we wanted.

The day I found myself browsing through that store was only a couple of months after I escaped from the worst relationship in my life. That day, in the midst of all of my heartache and worries of never finding anyone to love me, I stopped in front of the snow globe. Inside it was a peaceful glistening scene of a father decorating a Christmas tree in the woods with his two children—a little boy and a little girl. As I picked up the snow globe, tipped it upside down, and watched the puffy snow fall over my encapsulated dream, a passionate prayer murmured through my entire being: "God, please let me have a family someday."

After I brought the snow globe home, I made a habit of gazing into its magical world every night. Every night as I talked to God, I told him I trusted Him and that I knew as long as I was patient enough to wait for the right time, He'd give me the family I'd always dreamed of.

Once upon a time, I thought my life was over. I didn't think I would find anyone who'd ever really love me, or have a family of my own. I didn't have any friends. I wore drab-colored clothing, and when people saw me they often said my eyes looked empty and lifeless. I'd been so traumatized by some bad experiences that I was afraid I might never be able to live on my own or hold any kind of real job again.

But still, deep inside of me, flickers of hope and faith remained. Even on my loneliest, scariest days, I told myself that as long as I continued to trust in both God and myself, things would work out—somehow. I fought back the fears inside of me, and found a job and an apartment of my own. My snow globe came with me to that apartment. And as each difficult day passed, I continued to grow stronger. I began to wear vibrant colors, like fuchsia and lime green and dark purple. I discovered that I actually like to laugh a lot, and I made my first new friends in years. I stopped worrying that I would always be "alone," because I was finally happy. I felt beautiful and capable. And then, I met Todd—my best friend and biggest supporter, and now my husband.

The day I met Todd, I knew God would never let me down.

I won't always know all the answers to life's questions or know what the future holds, but I know that as long as I continue to trust God and myself, everything will always work out. It was only when I lacked faith and tried to control my own life that things went awry in the past: When I was too afraid of being alone to wait for the right person, I ended up being half of "that couple" who you could always hear screaming at each other through the walls of our apartment building. When I was too afraid of failing as a writer to actually stay at my computer and write, I began focusing on food and hating my body instead.

It wasn't until I finally learned to be patient and trusting that I started to get my life back on track.

Right now, my husband and I are living all the way across the country from our families. This is the first time I've ever lived farther than a hundred miles away from my parents. Because my husband is still in his (and our) journey through medical school, I don't know where we'll be living in two years, or four years, or eight years. But I do know that everything will be just fine.

Even though I'm not exactly living the life I always envisioned as a first grader, daydreaming in the back of my classroom (after all, I still don't have blonde hair or a red sports car!), these days I do *feel* the way I'd always imagined myself feeling as a grownup: peaceful, happy, and unconditionally loved.

Peace can come to anyone. You just have to learn to swim *with* the current of your life, instead of against it.

My never-ending prayer is that you will soon find peace in your life, too: No matter who you are, what you've gone through, or what your life is like today, you can turn everything around. It might not be easy and it certainly will take some time, but it *is* possible and it is worth every bit of the effort it will take to get there.

Open your eyes and your heart. Make some changes. Take the time, and have some faith: Go discover how truly amazing life can be!

CONTRIBUTORS

Adrienne, 23, California
Aleksandra, 32, Ontario
Alethia, 26, Arizona
Alexandra, 23, Sussex, England
Alicia Houston, 24, Illinois
Alison, 18, Vermont
Allie, 23, Pennsylvania
Ally, 20, Washington
Amy Pettengill, 27, New Hampshire
Amy Watson, 35, Connecticut
Andrea Roe, 28, British Columbia, Canada
Angela, 29, California
Anita, 41, Indiana
Annika, 19, California
Anthony, 31, Brighton, Great Britain
April, 16, Idaho
Arielle Lee Bair, 27, Pennsylvania
Ashley Devitt, 18, Florida
Barbara Murphy, Psy. D, 52, California
Bremandy, 34, Georgia
Brittany, 26, Maryland
Brooke, 34, California
Carolyn, 20, Ontario, Canada
Cassidy, 20, Pennsylvania
Cheryl, 49, Pennsylvania
Cheryl Kerrigan, 41, Massachusetts
Claire, 16, Connecticut
Dannielle, 23, Massachusetts
David, 41, Florida
Dawn, 16, Wisconsin
Deb K., 43, North Carolina
Delia, 32, New Jersey
Dr. Diana Repack, 46, Pennsylvania
E.B., 24, California
Elizabeth, 18, New York
Ellen, 26, New York
Heather, 18, New Hampshire
Heather, 36, Missouri
Hilary Crist, 27, California
Jan Lockert, 53, Ohio
Janis, 19, California
Jenni, 24, Texas
Jennifer, 30, Missouri
Jessica, 29, Texas
Jody Lanham, 55, Ohio
Julia, 23, Worcestershire, England
Kathy, 20, Utah
Kathy, 43, North Carolina
Kel, 23, Cheshire, England
Kelly, 18, New Jersey
Kelly, 28, New Jersey
Kelly Michaels, 39, Minnesota
Kristen, 25, Wisconsin
Kristy, 36, Arizona
Laura, 18, Tennesee
Laura R., 30, New York
Lauren B., 24, New York
Lindsey Wert, 24, California
Lisa, 30, Northern Ireland
Liz, 24, Florida
Lori, 30, Florida
Maria, 21, Mexico City, Mexico
Marie, 31, Fargo, North Dakota
Marisol, 20, California
Mary, 23, Wisconsin
Mary G., 49, Oregon
Maura, 18, Ohio
Meg, 16, Nottingham, England
Melissa, 21, Florida
Michelle M. S., 19, Mexico City, Mexico
Missy B., 34, Pennsylvania
Nicole, 19, Texas
Nicole Geddie, 24, New Mexico
Olivia, 30, Mississippi
Patrick Bergstrom, 26, Maryland
Rachel, 22, Ontario, Canada

Rachelle, 23, Arizona
Rayna, Psy.D, 26, Ohio
Russell Delderfield, 34, West Yorkshire, England
Samantha, 16, Ohio
Sarah, 30, Nevada
Savannah, 25, South Dakota
Shana, 24, Ohio
Shannon, 22, Texas
Sharon, 32, Nova Scotia, Canada
Sharon R Peterson, LCSW-C, 44, Maryland
Suzanne Yerdon Lewandowski, 55, Massachusetts
Rachael, MSW, Age XX, New York
Tara, 29, Michigan
Thecla, 24, Illinois
Tiffany, 26, Ohio
Traci, 37, California
Troy Roness, 23, North Dakota
Vicky Ann, 24, United Kingdom

RESOURCES

Websites

Justine Duppong website/blog:	http://youupcycled.com
Academy for Eating Disorders:	http://www.aedweb.org
Academy of Nutrition and Dietetics:	http://www.eatright.org
Andrea's Voice Foundation:	http://andreasvoice.org
Eating Disorder Referral and Information Center:	http://www.edreferral.com
Gurze Books:	http://www.bulimia.com
International Association of Eating Disorder Professionals:	http://www.iaedp.com
MentorConnect:	http://www.mentorconnect-ed.org
National Eating Disorders Association (NEDA):	http://www.nationaleatingdisorders.org
Something Fishy Website on Eating Disorders:	http://www.something-fishy.org
United States Department of Agriculture:	http://www.choosemyplate.gov/
Volunteer Match	http://www.volunteermatch.org/

Books

Chapman, Gary. *The 5 Love Languages: The Secret to Love that Lasts.* Chicago: Northfield Publishing, 2009.

Huebner, Dawn, and Matthews, Bonnie (Illustrator). *What to Do When You Worry Too Much: A Kid's Guide to Overcoming Anxiety (What to Do Guides for Kids).* Washington, DC: Magination Pr, 2005.

McKay, Matthew, Davis, Martha, and Fanning, Patrick. *Thoughts and Feelings: Taking Control of Your Moods and Your Life.* Oakland: New Harbinger, 2011.

Shannon, Marilyn M. *Fertility, Cycles, and Nutrition: Self-care for Improved Cycles and Fertility…Naturally!* 4th ed. Cincinnati: Couple to Couple League, 2009.

Wehrenberg, Margaret. *The 10 Best-Ever Anxiety Management Techniques.* New York: Norton, 2008.

Weschler, Toni. *Taking Charge of Your Fertility.* New York: HarperCollins, 2006.

ABOUT THE AUTHOR

Justine Duppong is an author, speaker, and coach, with education and experience in both counseling and health administration. She and her husband are the proud parents of two very sweet and spirited little girls. Visit Justine's blog at http://youupcycled.com.

Made in the USA
Las Vegas, NV
22 March 2026

44071332R00108